KT-171-946

The Organization of Maternity Care

A Guide to Evaluation

Edited by
Rona Campbell
and
Jo Garcia

Hochland & Hochland Ltd

Published by Hochland & Hochland Ltd, 174a Ashley Road, Hale, Cheshire, WA15 9SF, England.

© 1997, Rona Campbell and Jo Garcia

First edition

The cartoons in this book were drawn by Ros Asquith.

All rights reserved. No part of this book may be reproduced in any form or by any electronic or mechanical means, including information storage and retrieval systems, without permission in writing from the publisher, except by a reviewer who may quote brief passages in a review.

ISBN 1-898507-37-6

British Library Cataloguing in Publication Data
A catalogue record for this book is available from the British Library

Printed in Great Britain by Cromwell Press Ltd.

Contents

Contributors

Rona Campbell
Lecturer in Health Services Research, Department of Social Medicine, University of Bristol

Pam Dobson
Audit and Computer Liaison Midwife, Kings Healthcare Trust, London

Jo Garcia
Social Scientist, National Perinatal Epidemiology Unit, Oxford University

Alison Macfarlane
Medical Statistician, National Perinatal Epidemiology Unit, Oxford University

Nancy MacKeith
Midwife, Jahural Islam Medical College Hospital, Bhagalpur, Bangladesh

Miranda Mugford
Senior Lecturer, School of Health Policy and Practice, University of East Anglia

Mary Ness
Freelance researcher, Leeds

James Piercy
Research Fellow, York Health Economics Consortium

Jane Sandall
Reader in Midwifery, Department of Midwifery, City University, London.

Trudy Stevens
Researcher-Practitioner, Centre for Midwifery Practice, Thames Valley University and Hammersmith Hospitals NHS Trust

Acknowledgements

The editors would like to thank all the women, midwives and other staff who took part in the study that led up to this book. These people have to remain anonymous for reasons of confidentiality. This study was funded by the Department of Health and the National Health Service Executive.

Many people helped us with this book. Some undertook to read and comment on drafts of all, or parts of the book. Others provided useful information, suggested relevant literature or helped with the typing and editing of the numerous drafts. We are grateful to them all. In particular, we would like to thank:

Jean Ball – Saxilby, Lincolnshire.

Helen Betts – King Alfred College, Winchester.

Elizabeth Brandom – Royal College of Midwives, London.

Gill Craig – College of Health, London.

Rosemary Currell – Centre for Health Informatics, University of Wales, Aberystwyth.

Sue Dopson – Templeton College, Oxford University.

Tony Dowell – Centre for Research in Primary Care, University of Leeds.

Soo Downe, Jeanette Gilby – Derby City General Hospital.

Julie Grant – Birmingham Women's Health Care NHS Trust.

Christine Henderson – University of Central England, Birmingham.

Kate Jackson – Changing Childbirth Implementation Team.

Rosemary Johnson – Southmead Hospital, Bristol.

Hazel Ashurst, Sarah Ayers, Diana Elbourne, Natalie Kenney, Susan Law, Judith Lumley, Marie-Anne Martin and Siobhan Scanlan – National Perinatal Epidemiology Unit, Oxford.

Nick Mays – King's Fund Policy Institute, London.

Hazel McHaffie – University of Edinburgh.

Joan Greenwood, Jenny Griffin, Catherine Law, Jane McKessack, Kathryn Sallah and Rudi Singh – Department of Health, London.

Karin von Degenberg – NHS Executive, Leeds.

David Murray – Lambeth, Southark and Lewisham Health Authority, London.

Iris Neale, Julia Hares and Claire Diamond – Department of Social Medicine, University of Bristol.

Simon Plint – Beaumont Street Surgery, Oxford.

Mary Renfrew and Helene Price – Midwifery Studies, University of Leeds.

Noreen Shaw – Manor Hospital, Walsall.

Chris Sidgwick – South Warwickshire General Hospital NHS Trust

Jennifer Sleep – Thames Valley University.

Pat Strong and Jennifer Jones – Princess Margaret Hospital, Swindon.

Susan Thomas – Llandough Community Trust, Llandough Hospital, Penarth.

Ros Ullman – King's College, London.

Sarah Vause, Julie Wray and Angie Benbow – Royal College of Obstetricians and Gynaecologists Audit Unit, Manchester.

Patricia Weir – Rutherglen Maternity Hospital, Glasgow.

Foreword

The last three years have seen a great many changes in the way that maternity care is provided, not least in the philosophy underpinning it. However, there is more that can and should be done as we seek to implement the principles underlying Changing Childbirth.

Thorough planning before developments are carried out is vital to ensure success. This book will be an invaluable reference tool for anyone embarking on changes in the way that care is provided. It will help to ensure that those changes are fully evaluated not only for their impact on users, but also on those providing the service.

The editors have done a splendid job in putting such a comprehensive range of material together and I am sure that this will become an essential handbook for those seeking to improve maternity services for women and their families well into the 21st Century.

Julia Cumberlege.

BARONESS CUMBERLEGE
Chair of the Expert Maternity Group

CHAPTER ONE

Evaluating Maternity Care

Rona Campbell

The overall aim of this book is to give people who manage and provide maternity services a guide to enable them to evaluate existing and new ways of organizing maternity care. It is important to emphasize at the outset that the book is only concerned with the *organization* of maternity care, that is such things as team midwifery or providing individualized care. It does not deal with evaluating individual components of care, such as comparing different methods of managing the third stage of labour or investigating the effectiveness of postnatal pelvic floor exercises in preventing urinary incontinence. It is the view of the editors that new evaluations of the effectiveness of separate components of care should almost always be undertaken by randomized trials. While experimental methods have a place in the evaluation of maternity care organization, these do not necessarily answer all the questions that may be posed in an evaluation. This book therefore covers a wide range of techniques and methods.

There are ten chapters in the book and each is intended to fulfil one or two specific objectives. Although there is a logic to the way in which the chapters have been ordered, this is not really a book to be read from the first chapter to the last. Some ideas and examples recur in several chapters. The diagram on page 2 should help you to find your way round.

This first chapter introduces the book and looks at the need for evaluation. It also explains what evaluation is and how it is related to research and audit. In addition, it outlines the scope for evaluation, both in terms of issues in the organization of maternity care and the different directions that evaluations can take. Chapter 2 illustrates how to ensure that an evaluation is asking the right questions and takes the reader through the steps towards setting up such an evaluation.

The third chapter outlines the different methods that can be used to answer questions posed in an evaluation. Subsequent chapters then explore ways in which these methods can be used to evaluate the extent to which the goals of maternity services are being met. These chapters cover the various methods and techniques that can be employed when evaluating effectiveness and safety, the views of service users and service providers, service efficiency and sustainability.

Chapter 8 describes how NHS information systems can be used to support evaluations and Chapter 9 examines how simple evaluations can be achieved through audit. The final chapter, 'Planning an Evaluation', gives guidance on the practical tasks required before commencing an evaluation. It covers a diverse range from searching the literature to writing a research proposal. It also gives guidance on how much background work will be involved in evaluations of different degrees of complexity and scale.

Chapters in this book

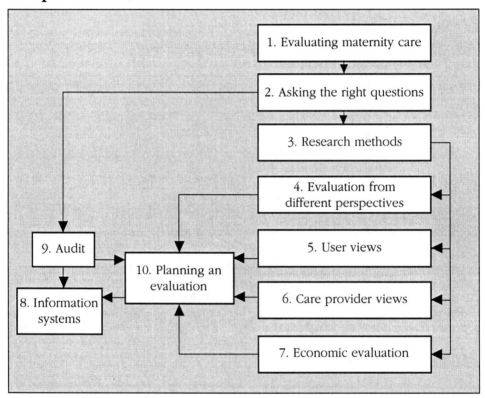

How should the book be used?

The most important requirement of anyone wanting to use this book is that they are interested in knowing the truth. It may be tempting to undertake or commission an evaluation simply to confirm beliefs. If the findings challenge these, a reaction can be to suppress the findings, or to denigrate the way in which the evaluation was done. At the outset of an evaluation there is nothing wrong with having an opinion as to which method of organization you think is best. What is wrong, is to allow such an opinion to bias the way in which the evaluation is undertaken, or not to accept findings which are contrary to expectations.

The people involved in writing this book have been actively engaged in the evaluation of different aspects of maternity care for many years. We have tried to approach the book with an understanding of the constraints that can make evaluations difficult and have thus tried to offer practical guidance as to how to achieve the best evaluations possible, with whatever resources are available. We have concentrated on evaluation at the local rather than national level. Most of the work at national level is carried out by specialist research organizations and government departments. In order to ground this book in practical reality, wherever possible we have given real examples from existing work to illustrate suggestions made in the text. The extent to which we have achieved our aims is for you to judge.

Why evaluate?

'New patterns of service should be designed to allow evaluation of both their effectiveness and their acceptability to women using the service.' (Department of Health, 1993)

During the last decade, the health service in Great Britain has undergone an unprecedented period of change. This began in the early 1980s with a series of piecemeal initiatives, such as the introduction of general management and the contracting out of certain ancillary services, which were introduced to try to improve efficiency and curb costs (Department of Health and Social Security, 1983). The more far-reaching structural changes were indicated in the government white paper *Working for Patients* published in 1989 (Department of Health, 1989). The core of these changes has been the introduction of an internal market in health care necessitating a separation between the purchasers of health care (health authorities) and the providers of hospital and community services. Many providers of these services have become self-governing trusts and general practitioners now have the opportunity to manage their own budgets and purchase services on behalf of their patients.

As well as these fundamental changes in the organization of the health service, national policy on maternity care has been transformed. This began with an enquiry into maternity services by the House of Commons Health Committee. In its report, the Health Committee signalled a significant departure from the policies advocated by many previous committees of enquiry when it noted that: 'Given the absence of conclusive evidence, it is no longer acceptable that the pattern of maternity care provision should be driven by presumptions about the applicability of a medical model of care based on unproven assertions' (House of Commons Health Committee, 1992). It went on to recommend many changes, including real choice about place of birth, greater emphasis on continuity of care and enhanced professional autonomy for midwives which, with the publication of *Changing Childbirth* (Department of Health, 1993), and its subsequent acceptance by the government (Department of Health, 1994) have now become official policy. Similar policy documents were prepared in Scotland and Northern Ireland (Scottish Office Home and Health Department, 1992; Maternity Unit Study Group, 1994). As a result of these policy developments, and the wider reorganizations within the health service, there is considerable pressure for change in the organization of maternity care. While this has generated a good deal of excitement about the possibility of extending and developing new ways of delivering services, it has also produced concern that things which worked well in the past may be sacrificed in the enthusiasm to be seen to be offering different and progressive forms of care.

The history of maternity care provides many examples of well intentioned changes which were not fully evaluated before their widespread introduction. Some of these were found later to be ineffective, for example, antenatal breast shells for inverted or flat nipples, or occasionally, as in the case of diethylstilboestrol, tragically harmful (Enkin et al., 1995). Paradoxically, history also demonstrates how difficult it can be to ensure widespread use of effective treatments and models of care, even when evidence of how well they work has been published in prominent places (Department of Health, 1993).

Evaluations of new forms of maternity care are needed for many reasons. Firstly, new ways of organizing care, introduced to improve the service, can have unintended consequences. For example, a satellite clinic for 'disadvantaged' women may improve the continuity of care that women get, but may be experienced as stigmatizing because of staff attitudes (Reid et al., 1983). Expectations can also be unrealistic and carers and clients may feel keen disappointment with a new service (Stewart, 1995). Another danger is that new schemes may lead to the loss of existing successful forms of care. The introduction of team midwifery, for instance, has led to the demise of domino deliveries in some areas (Wardle et al., 1997). In a new scheme the use of resources can also be difficult to predict. Travel or equipment costs, or staff overtime may exceed expectations. Finally, the planned pattern of care may not be achieved in practice, or may not be achieved for some women, or for some aspects of the service. In these situations changes can appear to make little difference to women or staff (Currell, 1990).

As the quote at the beginning of this section illustrates, it is now a requirement of maternity service policy that changes to the service be evaluated. While few would disagree with this, many of those wishing to introduce change feel apprehensive about evaluation and are afraid that they do not have the knowledge, skill or resources at their disposal to carry it out properly. Tangible evidence of this is the large number of enquiries to bodies like the Changing Childbirth Implementation Team and National Perinatal Epidemiology Unit (NPEU), from those seeking help and guidance with a huge variety of evaluations.

It is foolish to suggest that all aspects of the organization of maternity care be subject to constant evaluation but often the reasons given for failing to evaluate can be spurious, as Box 1.1 suggests.

Recognizing the need for more developmental work on evaluation of midwifery care organization, the Department of Health, when *Changing Childbirth* (Department of Health, 1993) was published, also invited tenders from organizations who could assist three midwifery service providers with evaluations. In its tender the NPEU identified the need to provide some detailed guidance for those wishing to evaluate aspects of the organization of maternity care. The tender submitted by the NPEU was successful and this book is one of the results of that project.

Box 1.1: To evaluate or not to evaluate

Reasons for not wanting to evaluate:

1. *Already enough evidence that this scheme works*
   This is a good reason for not undertaking large scale research but local implementation of a new way of delivering care may well require evaluation.

2. *No time – got to get this new scheme off the ground otherwise we'll lose the money for it*
   Evaluations don't have to be elaborate and take months of planning. An audit of routine data collected before and after the introduction of a new scheme is better than no evaluation. Good managers should want to know what is happening.

3. *No money*
   Even if there is no additional money for evaluation, audit should still be an option.

4. *Don't need to evaluate – it's obviously working well*
   Opinion is no substitute for evidence.

5. *Don't want to evaluate this*
   Providing and managing a service carries with it a responsibility to ensure that what is provided is what is needed.

Evaluation, audit and research: what is the difference?

Evaluation, audit and research are distinguished by the aims of those undertaking these activities rather than by the methods used, which in many instances can be the same. Precisely how research, audit and evaluation should be defined is the subject of much academic debate. Rather than engage in such a debate, we have tried to provide a simple description of the major characteristics of the three activities in order to distinguish them.

Evaluation

Dictionary definitions of the verb 'to evaluate' suggest that it is simply to find the value of something, in other words finding out if something is useful, if it works as intended. Any foray into the literature on maternity care or conversation with those working in the field, however, tends to indicate that the word evaluation has a variety of different uses and meanings.

Many are familiar with the 'evaluation form' handed out at the end of a meeting or conference asking for feedback on everything, from the ease of finding the venue, to the quality of the speakers. This notion of evaluation as feedback appears to be quite common, particularly in relation to service users (Jones et al., 1987). The word 'evaluation' is also used interchangeably with words such as 'appraisal' and 'assessment' or phrases such as 'critical review' (Marnoch, 1992). The word evaluation is also used to describe studies in which new schemes are judged against some kind of criterion, whether it is a control group (i.e. a group which has not been dealt with under the new scheme), previous practice (Twaddle et al., 1993), agreed good practice or policy guidelines (Williams et al., 1989) or research evidence.

While there appears to be a discrepancy between the simple definition of evaluation offered in many English dictionaries and its more complex use in health services literature, such a difference does not in reality exist. All of the studies cited above were attempting to find out how valuable or useful something was. The difference lies not in the intention but the approach taken.

Broadly speaking there are two approaches to evaluation. The first is essentially subjective and involves seeking views and ideas as to whether or not something is of value. In its most unsophisticated form this is feedback. The second approach attempts to be objective by comparing a system of delivering maternity care with some predetermined criteria. It is this second approach to evaluation which is embodied in the WHO definition of evaluation: 'the systematic and scientific process of determining the extent to which an action or set of actions was successful in the achievement of pre-determined objectives' (Royal College of Physicians of London, 1989).

Audit

Many people think of an audit as external scrutiny of financial accounts to check that a proper record of all transactions has been kept and that 'the books balance'. This type of audit does take place in the health service. More commonly, though, 'audit' is used to mean clinical audit. Clinical audit means reviewing the way in which health care is delivered to find out if what should be happening, is happening. If deficiencies are identified, then audit may also involve putting remedies into place, and repeating the auditing process to see if change has occurred.

One of the earliest examples of a clinical audit is the system of *Confidential Enquiries into Maternal Deaths*, which is still functioning. There were many reports produced on maternal mortality in the early part of the century, including several by the Ministry of Health, reflecting the widespread concern about the high maternal death toll (Campbell and Macfarlane, 1994). In 1952, however, following a reorganization within the Ministry of Health, a voluntary, standardized system of data collection on all maternal deaths was put in place. This enabled reviews to be undertaken by panels of independent assessors in which it was possible to identify areas where care was deficient and deaths could be avoided. One early result of this process of auditing was the introduction of a comprehensive network of obstetric flying squads because the absence of prompt treatment for women with retained placentae, following birth at home, was identified as major cause of preventable maternal mortality (Crombie et al., 1993).

Audit can thus be considered one approach to evaluation. If the aims of a maternity scheme can be specified, and these aims translated into measurable objectives, then it is possible to undertake a basic audit to determine if the service is achieving its goals. For example, if one of the service aims is to provide continuity of carer, then a count can be made of the number of different members of staff a defined group of women came into contact with during the time they were being cared for by the service. This particular approach to evaluation has been used in studies of continuity of carer (Thomson, 1991).

Research

The purpose of research is to generate new knowledge and to answer questions which have hitherto remained unanswered. It is thus possible to make a clear distinction between research and audit, 'the difference is between adding to the body of medical knowledge and ensuring that knowledge is effectively used' (Crombie et al., 1993). Scientific knowledge often accumulates slowly. Many pieces of research on the same topic may be required before something can be said to be scientific fact. An example of this is the knowledge that we now have of the advantages of women in labour having a trained support person with them continuously. A whole series of experimental research studies, undertaken in a variety of different settings, have consistently shown that having a trained support person with a woman throughout active labour reduced the likelihood of medication for pain, of instrumental delivery, of caesarean section and of five minute Apgar scores under seven (Hodnett, 1994).

Most evaluations do not therefore constitute research because the primary aim is not to generate new knowledge but rather to test whether existing knowledge is being applied appropriately and successfully.

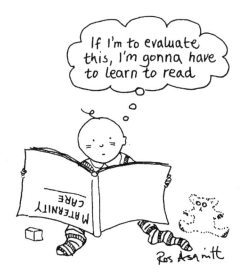

What focuses can an evaluation take?

If 'to evaluate' means to determine whether or not something is of value, then an obvious problem is deciding what is 'of value' when providing maternity care. One way of looking at this is to consider what 'values' underpin or should underpin the provision of publicly funded maternity care in the United Kingdom. Put another way, one could ask 'what are the key aims of the service?'. The 'Principles of Good Maternity

Care' set out at the beginning of *Changing Childbirth* and reproduced below offer a starting point.

> 'The woman must be the focus of maternity care. She should be able to feel that she is in control of what is happening to her and be able to make decisions about her care, based on her needs, having discussed the matter fully with the professionals involved.
>
> Maternity services must be readily and easily accessible to all. They should be sensitive to the needs of the local population and based primarily in the community.
>
> Women should be involved in the monitoring and planning of maternity services to ensure they are responsive to the needs of a changing society. In addition care should be effective and resources used efficiently.' (Department of Health, 1993)

These principles can be amplified and extended into five key goals for maternity care. It should aim to be:

1. Effective and safe for the women and their babies who use it, and for the staff who provide it;
2. Acceptable to women and their families and sensitive to their needs;
3. Sustainable;
4. Efficient in its use of human and financial resources; and
5. Accessible to all and provided on an equitable basis.

Another approach to defining 'value' is to ask 'of value to whom?'. There are three candidates – users, providers and the wider society. The first is maternity service users. Providing 'women centred' maternity care is now part of official maternity care policy. Ensuring this is being achieved can only be done by seeking the views of the women and families who use the service. There is also increasing recognition that systems of care will only work well if those providing that care are happy and feel their professional skills are being put to good use. Seeking the views of care givers is thus an important approach whether an existing or new pattern of care is being evaluated. Finally, the value of any pattern of care in terms of its cost to the public purse and its contribution to the public good is another important area of evaluation.

What is there to be evaluated?

The purpose of this section is to chart the scope for evaluation by considering the major issues in the organization of maternity care. Precisely how to evaluate new forms of maternity care, introduced to address these issues, will be covered in later chapters.

The issue which has probably dominated the debate about the way in which maternity care should be organized more than any other is that of safety. Ensuring safe care continues to be a key goal of maternity services but it is now generally acknowledged that 'Used as an over-riding principle (*it*) may become an excuse for unnecessary interventions and technological surveillance which detract from the experience of the mother' and that 'It is important that benefits are proven rather than assumed' (Department of Health, 1993). Although intervention is specifically mentioned here, it is also the case that the way in which maternity care is organized also needs to be proven to be safe.

An example of an aspect of the organization of maternity care where enhancing safety has been assumed rather than demonstrated is antenatal care. While it has been shown that the treatment of specific complications arising during the antenatal period can be effective, it has still not been established whether or not routine antenatal care is of benefit to all and in particular to women likely to have uncomplicated pregnancies (Pearson, 1994). Clearly, only very large evaluations can address the issue of whether routine antenatal care does more good than harm, but there is still considerable scope for evaluating the organization of antenatal care in terms of the timing and frequency of visits, the relative merits of the various settings in which care can be provided, who provides the care (midwife, GP or obstetrician) and how accessible and acceptable it is. One trial comparing a reduction in the frequency of antenatal visits for women receiving shared antenatal care has recently been completed (Sikorski et al., 1996), as has a multi-centred trial to compare antenatal care provided by GPs and midwives with traditional shared care (Tucker et al., 1996).

The 'continued attendance of a midwife on the mother and baby' (UKCC, 1993) for a minimum of ten days after childbirth is a key feature of maternity care in the United Kingdom which is enshrined in statute. The purpose of these visits is to care for and support women with a new baby, often providing a bridge between hospital care and home. There has not been a great deal of work evaluating the extent to which the pattern of care provided meets the needs of women and their new-born babies (Garcia, Renfrew and Marchant, 1994). The traditional interpretation of the midwives' rule governing the postnatal period has been that 'continued attendance' meant that mothers must be visited at least once every day for ten days, although in more recent years a less rigid approach has been taken. One evaluation of a change to a more flexible pattern of postnatal visiting based on the perceived needs of individual women is discussed at greater length in Chapter 3 (Twaddle et al., 1993).

The concept of 'women centred care' is now firmly embedded in maternity care policy. There are at least two aspects to this; firstly giving women choice and enabling them to feel in control, and secondly meeting the needs of women as individuals. In trying to achieve more 'women centred care', it is recommended that every woman be given the name of a midwife to whom she can refer throughout her pregnancy. In addition, women are to be given the choice of the professional they wish to lead their care and an informed choice about where to give birth (Department of Health, 1993). There is obvious scope for a range of evaluations of these policies from simple audits to assess the extent to which they have been implemented, to evaluations of users' and providers' views of their worth. An evaluation of 'one-to-one midwifery practice' which is intended to provide 'sensitive, individual care, based on the unique needs and choices of women' has just been completed in a large London teaching hospital (McCourt and Page, 1996). An evaluation of a new maternity service in Nottingham entitled 'partners in care', which offers women a choice of four different packages of care from home birth through to total hospital care, is also underway (Pitman, 1996).

While all women have different individual needs some women have needs which may require additional resources. Firstly, there are women who have special medical and obstetric needs. The extent to which these groups of women, who often have very medicalized pregnancies, receive women-centred care is an area which requires evaluation (Thomas, 1996). Secondly, there are women who have 'average' medical and obstetric needs but require extra assistance if they are not to miss out on the maternity services that are available. An example of an evaluation in this field is one based in the Yorkshire Region to assess the quality of the maternity services for Muslim women from Pakistan and indigenous white women (Hirst and Hewison, 1995).

Continuity of care, and in particular continuity of carer, have been identified as key factors in making pregnancy and childbirth a positive experience (House of Commons Health Committee, 1992). While there is good evidence from randomized trials to show that continuity of companion in labour improves outcome it has not, however, been shown to be beneficial when applied to the whole of maternity care (Enkin et al., 1995). One of the main organizational responses to trying to achieve greater continuity of care has been the introduction of team midwifery. A detailed study of this by Wraight and colleagues (1993) showed that, while over a third of maternity units in England and Wales claimed to be using some form of team midwifery, there was no consensus as to what constituted team midwifery. The researchers reported that only a third of the team midwifery schemes established in the five years preceding the study had been evaluated and likewise only a third of those schemes which had been discontinued had been subject to any evaluation. Where evaluations had been undertaken these appeared to have consisted largely of obtaining 'feedback' (in other words reactions of staff and users) rather than any systematic attempt to compare the new schemes with previous systems of care. Only a small minority of evaluations had involved any auditing of clinical care or economic appraisal. Given the continuing emphasis on continuity of carer in current policy, further evaluations of team midwifery from a whole range of perspectives are needed.

Scope also exists for evaluation of the different ways in which maternity, and in particular, midwifery services are managed. Comparing integrated midwifery services with those where the management of those working in hospital and community trusts is separate is just one example.

A concern about the introduction of new forms of maternity care is the extent to which they can be sustained in the long term. New schemes may be introduced because of the enthusiasm of one individual or a small group of particularly committed staff who are very determined to make it work and who, in their enthusiasm, may work in a way which cannot be sustained. The way in which groups of women should be allocated to midwives, the optimum number of women for which an individual midwife or group of midwives can care, taking into account the level of need among the women, are all issues which are subject to a great deal of debate and which need to be addressed in evaluations of caseload, team and group midwifery practice.

The final objective listed in *Changing Childbirth* is that 'the service provided must represent value for money and the cost and benefit of alternative arrangements assessed locally' (Department of Health, 1993). Considerable opportunity exists for evaluating the costs of new forms of maternity care. For example, it is sometimes assumed that the saving in cost is one of the benefits which will accrue from a change to midwifery-led care. A randomized trial comparing women giving birth in a midwife-led unit with those giving birth in the adjacent consultant unit, which included an economic appraisal, found that establishing a separate midwifery-led unit resulted in a significant rise in the cost per woman (Hundley et al., 1995). This rise was due in part to the different gradings for the midwives employed in the two settings.

In the 1970s concern grew about whether the move from home to hospital birth, and the trend towards the active management of labour, was resulting in an erosion of the role of the midwife. A study of midwives, health visitors, general practitioners and obstetric medical staff showed that while midwives provided the majority of maternity care, a substantial proportion were not able to utilize their full range of skills or exercise the degree or responsibility for which they had been trained (Robinson, Golden and Bradley, 1983). A more recent study looked at the impact on the work of both midwives and medical practitioners of not having registrars on the labour ward. Midwives working on wards without registrars enjoyed higher levels of job satisfaction but there was more likely to be conflict with senior house officers. Consultants working on wards without registrars tended to have a positive attitude towards midwives and were more likely to see themselves as 'practitioners' rather than 'managers' (Green et al., 1990). Further scope exists for investigating skill mix both between and within professional groups.

There is increasing recognition of the need to evaluate the impact of new forms of maternity care on those providing that care as well as those receiving it. An example of this approach was taken when a midwifery development unit was established with midwives aiming to provide total care throughout pregnancy and childbirth. Questionnaires were issued to all midwives prior to the inception of the new unit and again after the unit had been functioning for 15 months. Midwives attached to the development unit experienced significant positive change in attitudes and there was no evidence of increased levels of stress. No change was recorded in the attitudes of midwives who continued their usual pattern of work and were not part of the development unit (Turnbull et al., 1995). There is also a need to consider how changes in midwifery might affect the work of other staff in the maternity services and more widely (see Chapter 6).

Principles for evaluating maternity care

At the outset of this chapter it was made clear that this book is concerned with evaluating the way in which maternity care is organized and not with individual components of care. Many of the individual components of care given during pregnancy and childbirth have been the subject of a systematic review. Such reviews are published in an electronic form, which is regularly updated, in the relevant reviews within the Cochrane Library (see Chapter 10). In the second edition of a shorter written guide to this evidence (Enkin et al., 1995), the principles by which the editors judge whether certain forms of care are beneficial or not are set out. They are:

- The only justification for practices that restrict a women's autonomy, her freedom of choice, and her access to her baby, would be clear evidence that these restrictive practices do more good than harm.

- Any interference with the natural process of pregnancy and childbirth should also be shown to do more good than harm.

- The onus of proof rests on those who advocate any intervention that interferes with either of these principles.

While these principles were formulated for judging evidence relating to interventions in pregnancy and childbirth, they could apply equally well to evaluations of the organization of maternity care. These are principles which the editors of this book endorse and would commend to readers.

In subsequent chapters the methods used in some of the studies mentioned here will be described in detail to illustrate the range of methods that can be used. The next chapter describes some of the preliminary steps that need to be undertaken in initiating an evaluation.

References

Campbell, R., Macfarlane, A. (1994). *Where to Be Born?* Second Edition. Oxford: National Perinatal Epidemiology Unit.

Crombie, I.K., Davies, H.T.O., Abraham, S.C.S., Florey, C.duV. (1993). *The Audit Handbook.* Chichester: Wiley.

Currell, R. (1990). 'The organization of midwifery care'. In: Alexander, J., Levy, V., Roch, S. (Eds). *Antenatal Care. A Research Based Approach.* Basingstoke: Macmillan.

Department of Health (1994). *Women Will Have A Greater Say in Maternity Care: Mother and Baby Come First.* Press release 93/94. Jan 24. London: Department of Health.

Department of Health and Social Security (1983). *Competitive Tendering in the Provision of Domestic, Catering and Laundry Services.* HC (83)18, London: DHSS.

Department of Health, Welsh Office, Scottish Home and Health Department and Northern Ireland Office (1989). *Working for Patients.* CM 555. London: HMSO.

Department of Health (1993). *Changing Childbirth.* Part I. Report of the Expert Maternity Group. London: HMSO.

Enkin, M., Keirse, M.J.C.N., Renfrew, M., Neilson, J. (1995). *A Guide to Effective Care in Pregnancy and Childbirth.* Oxford: Oxford University Press.

Garcia, J., Renfrew, M., Marchant, S. (1994). 'Postnatal home visiting by midwives'. *Midwifery,* Vol. 10, pp. 40–43.

Green, J.V., Green, J.M., Coupland V.A. (1990). 'Labour relations: Doctors and midwives on the labour ward'. In: Garcia, J., Kilpatrick, R., Richards, M. (Eds). *The Politics of Maternity Care.* Oxford: Oxford University Press.

Hirst, J., Hewison, J. (1995). 'Assessing the quality of the maternity services for Muslim women from Pakistan and indigenous white women. Evaluating maternity services seminar'. 13th February, London: King's Fund.

Hodnett, E.D. (1994). 'Support from caregivers during childbirth'. In: Enkin, M., Keirse M., Renfrew, M., Neilson, J. (Eds). *Cochrane Database of Systematic Reviews.* Review No 03871, Oxford: Update Software.

House of Commons Health Committee (1992). *Maternity Services.* Vol I, report. (Chairman N Winterton). HC 29-I. London: HMSO.

Hundley, V.A., Donaldson, C., Lang, G.D. et al. (1995). 'Costs of intrapartum care in a midwife-managed unit and a consultant led labour ward'. *Midwifery*, Vol. 11, pp. 103–109.

Jones, L., Leneman, L., Maclean, U. (1987). *Consumer Feedback for the NHS: A Literature Review*. London: King's Fund.

Marnoch, A. (1992). 'An evaluation of the importance of formal, maternal fetal movement counting as a measure of fetal well-being'. *Midwifery*, Vol. 8, No. 2, pp. 54–69.

Maternity Unit Study Group (1994). *Delivering Choice*. Belfast: Department of Health and Social Services.

McCourt, C., Page, L. (Eds.) (1996). *Report on the Evaluation of One to One Midwifery Practice*. London: The Hammersmith Hospitals NHS Trust & Thames Valley University.

Pearson, V. (1994). *Frequency and Timing of Antenatal Visits*. Bristol: Health Care Evaluation Unit, University of Bristol.

Pitman, A. (1996). 'Nottingham's pregnancy diary project'. *Changing Childbirth Update*, No. 5, p. 9.

Reid, M., McIlwaine, G., Gutteridge, S. (1983). *A Comparison of the Delivery of Antenatal Care between a Hospital and a Peripheral Clinic*. Glasgow: University of Glasgow Social Paediatric and Obstetric Research Unit.

Robinson, S., Golden, J., Bradley, S. (1983). *A Study of the Role and Responsibilities of the Midwife*. NERU Report No. 1, Nursing Education Research Unit, London: Kings College, London University.

Royal College of Physicians of London, Working Party on Medical Audit (1989). *Medical Audit: A First Report: What Why and How?* London: Royal College of Physicians of London.

Scottish Office Home and Health Department (1992). *Provision of Maternity Services in Scotland. A Policy Review*. Edinburgh: Scottish Office Home and Health Department.

Sikorski, J., Wilson, J., Clement, S. et al. (1996). 'A randomized controlled trial comparing two schedules of antenatal visits: the antenatal care project'. *BMJ*, Vol. 312, pp. 546–53.

Stewart, M. (1995). 'Do you have to know your midwife?'. *British Journal of Midwifery*, Vol. 3, pp. 19–20.

Thomas, H. (1996). *Major Illness During Pregnancy: Women's Views*. Occasional Paper. Department of Sociology, Guildford: University of Surrey.

Thomson, A.M. (1991). 'Providing care at a midwives' antenatal clinic'. In: Robinson, S., Thomson, A.M. (Eds). *Midwives, Research and Childbirth 2*. London: Chapman and Hall.

Tucker, J.S., Hall, P., Howie, P.W. et al. (1996). 'Should obstetricians see women with normal pregnancies? A multi centred randomised controlled trial of routine antenatal care led by general practitioners and midwives compared with shared care led by obstetricians'. *BMJ*, Vol. 312, pp. 554–59.

Turnbull, D., Reid, M., McGinley, M., Sheilds N.R. (1995). 'Changes in midwives' attitudes to their professional role following the implementation of the midwifery development unit'. *Midwifery*, Vol. 11, pp. 110–119.

Twaddle, S., Liao, X.H., Fyvie, H. (1993). 'An evaluation of postnatal care individualised to the needs of the women'. *Midwifery*, Vol. 9, No. 3, pp. 154–160.

UKCC (1993). *Midwives Rules*. London: United Kingdom Central Council for Nursing, Midwifery and Health Visiting.

Wardle, S., Wright, P.J., Court, B.V. (1997). 'Knowledge and preference for the domino delivery option'. *Midwifery* (Forthcoming).

Williams, S., Dickson, D., Forbes, J. et al. (1989). 'An evaluation of community antenatal care'. *Midwifery*, Vol. 5, No. 2, pp. 63–68.

Wraight, A., Ball, J., Seccombe, I., Stock, J. (1993). *Mapping Team Midwifery*. Institute of Manpower Studies, Report Series 242, Brighton: IMS.

CHAPTER TWO

Asking The Right Questions

Jo Garcia and Rona Campbell

Before starting an evaluation it is important to give some thought to the question or questions that you are trying to answer. This chapter explores practical ways of ensuring that your evaluation is asking the right questions. How to go about answering those questions is covered in Chapters 3 to 7 where different research methods are described and discussed. The work you put in at this stage will be crucial and should ensure that the evaluation is well focused and has an appropriate design. This, in turn, will increase the chances that it will be taken seriously by decision makers when it is complete.

Questions about maternity care

In the first chapter we suggested that maternity care should be:

- Effective and safe
- Acceptable to women and families
- Sustainable
- Efficient
- Equitable.

In this chapter we consider how these goals can be translated into specific questions which might form the basis of an evaluation. The groups of questions are intended as examples and not as complete lists. We then go on to describe the practical steps that can be taken to ensure that your evaluation gets off to a good start.

Effective and safe

The main question under this heading is: do the different ways of organizing care lead to different outcomes for mothers and babies? In practice, though, we need to split this question up and look at specific aspects of care and particular outcomes. Here are some examples of questions that we could ask about the safety and effectiveness of care:

- Does the presence of a known care giver in labour reduce the need for pain relief in labour or improve breastfeeding success or lead to other good outcomes for mother and baby?

- Does a reduction in the number of antenatal visits with a consultant obstetrician lead to an increase in undiagnosed pregnancy complications?
- Does a special counselling service reduce the negative impact of perinatal bereavement on parents?

Evaluations which have attempted to address questions of safety and effectiveness are discussed further in Chapter 4.

Acceptable to women and families

The general question to be asked is: what are the views, experiences and preferences of service users? More specifically we could ask:

- What does it mean to 'know' your midwife?
- What role do women want the GP to play in their maternity care?
- What sorts of conflicting advice are a problem for women?

Women's reactions to their care are often explored in studies that evaluate different models of care. Many local studies have asked women to provide information for audit, for example, by finding out whether they knew their care givers in labour or were given advice about particular things. Studies have also looked at whether women consider that the services are meeting their needs, for example, whether care is accessible to them and whether they are interested in new services like drop-in clinics or locally based care. There have been national sample surveys to look at the key issues for women receiving maternity care and to help with policy making. Specific examples of how users' views have been investigated are described and discussed in Chapter 5.

Sustainable

A pattern of care is sustainable if the human and financial resources needed to set it up, and make it work in the longer-term, are likely to be available. When we are exploring alternative models of provision we need to ask what benefits they provide, what they cost, who bears the cost in the short and long term and what implications they have for the work and skills of care givers in the short and long term. Some typical questions include:

- How much do alternative patterns of care cost, over time, and who bears the cost?
- Do improved outcomes achieved justify any extra cost?
- What are the implications of different models of care for staff training, retention and development?
- Are there good ways of introducing and sustaining new ways of working?

In practice this means research in two main areas: economic evaluation of the new models of care and studies of the views and careers of staff. Health economics is a rapidly growing field and now more studies in health services include an economic component. Chapter 7 deals with economic evaluation in maternity care in greater detail and Chapter 6 discusses how to assess the impact of changes on staff.

Efficient

Efficiency is not about outcomes but is about practical and sensible ways of providing the service, although care cannot be considered truly efficient if it is not effective. It is about good communication and record keeping, following agreed policies, not making women wait a long time at a clinic, avoiding duplication, not losing records, cutting down on the numbers of forms that staff have to fill in, or not asking women to come to the hospital on a separate occasion for blood samples to be taken. Examples of specific questions include:

- Are the goals of care explicit and is there a way of knowing whether or not the goals are being met?
- Is there unnecessary duplication of work?
- Is communication effective?
- Are information systems useful and reliable?
- Can record keeping be made less time consuming for staff?

Once a form of care is shown to be effective, then how can it be provided efficiently in particular local circumstances? There are no absolutes about efficiency because the best ways of doing things are affected by specific local needs and resources. Chapter 8 is about local maternity information systems and how they can be used in evaluation and Chapter 9 is about approaches to audit. There are also other types of study that lead to information about efficiency such as financial reviews, studies of record keeping and handling, studies of travel and time use, and more descriptive studies where a researcher collects information by observing what is taking place.

Accessible and equitable

Some of the issues to be addressed under this heading are:

- Are some women excluded from care because they cannot afford to get to the place of care?
- What provision is made for women who do not speak English?
- Does the quality of care vary substantially between providers or for categories of women within a provider unit?
- Are some types of care luxuries?

Should we look at equity only in terms of parity of funding? What if some women or some communities have needs that make their care more expensive in the short term, even if in the longer term money may be saved? Women who do not speak English cannot have acceptable care without access to interpreting, and studies show that many do not. By emphasizing access to care we can help to justify special provision for those who need it – interpreters, drop in clinics, home visits, teams with special areas of responsibility and so on. Looked at another way, the issue of targeting of care is also one of equity. For example, is it particularly valuable to offer home antenatal visits to particular women, or categories of women? Should longer hospital stays be available to those who want them, or recommended (as at present) to women who have had a difficult delivery, or some other problem? Overall, there has been little evaluation of the changes in service organization from the point of view of appropriate targeting of care, accessibility of care for certain groups or the equitable distribution of resources.

Much of the evaluation of maternity services in relation to equity has to be done at a national level and is therefore not within the scope of this book. Moreover, many of the questions raised under this heading are not to be addressed simply by research. They concern moral positions where opinions vary. Evaluation can supply information to make the debates more useful, but political and moral judgements will be crucial.

Having described in some detail what sort of questions might be asked when evaluating whether maternity services are meeting their overall goals we now review some practical steps which may help identify the aims and objectives of specific local services and help to clarify what questions your evaluation should be asking.

Your current service: describing what is and how it came into being

A useful first step in any evaluation is to compile a description of the service and you may also want to include in this an account of how it came into being. Begin your description with where the service is located (e.g. teaching hospital, domiciliary, health centre) then give details of the staff who provide it (e.g. numbers, grades and whole time equivalents), the characteristics of the population it serves (e.g. birth rate, age structure, family size, social economic composition, whether rural or urban), how many women use the service and how it relates to other hospital and primary care services. You also need to try and look at the care it provides from the point of view of the women who use it, for example, by indicating what choices it affords them.

Compiling such a description will involve acquiring routine statistics about service activity, the staff employed and the population served. Public health departments in purchaser organizations should be able to provide details about the population served and personnel and information departments of provider units should be able to supply the other data.

Describing how the service came into being, how it has developed and how it currently operates in relation to other services may require you to interview some key informants, and read papers and the minutes of meetings at which the service was discussed. For example, imagine you wanted to evaluate a DOMINO scheme which has been in operation in the maternity unit of your district general hospital for the last ten years. The current impression is that the numbers of women using the service has been declining in the last year or so and there is some suggestion that maybe it should be stopped.

Supposing you have assembled the routine data and these show that numbers using the scheme have declined, although this is part of a general fall in the birth rate in the locality. You are now trying to find out why the service began. You have only been working at the maternity unit for five years so you decide to interview a retired senior midwife and obstetrician, both of whom worked at the unit when the DOMINO service began, a community midwife who has worked on the district since before the service began and who still regularly brings women into the unit under the scheme, a local GP obstetrician whose practice uses the DOMINO scheme and a local National Childbirth Trust antenatal teacher who has worked in the area for the last 15 years.

It turns out that some of your key informants were on a working party set up by the local district health authority to advise on whether such a service should be introduced. They point to where some of the papers from this may be and having tracked them down you find that they indicate one of the prime reasons for setting up the service was to try to stop women having home births; most of the obstetricians and some of the local GPs at the time were very opposed to them. It appears that many of the community midwives wished to undertake home births but they were persuaded that the DOMINO scheme was a better option.

As the hypothetical example above illustrates, compiling such a description can begin to clarify some of the questions that the evaluation should address. In this instance how much of the decline in use in the DOMINO scheme was just a reflection of a more general decline in the birth rate? Also, if the decline was real could it be because women and midwives preferred birth at home to the DOMINO scheme and the advent of the policy initiative *Changing Childbirth* had made this a real choice again?

Defining the aims and objectives of your service

Having described your service the next essential step is to list what it is trying to achieve in the form of its aims and objectives. A key aspect of any evaluation is to examine the extent to which service aims and objectives are being met. To proceed without having established what the aims and objectives of the services are, will render the evaluation meaningless. Consultation with all those involved in the provision of the service will be required in drawing up aims and objectives. This may take some time and involve considerable negotiation.

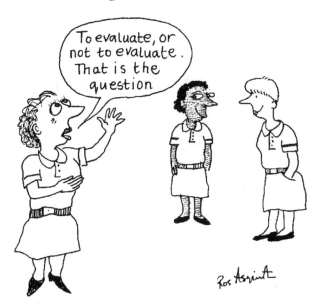

Box 2.1 gives a set of aims for an imaginary service for women with complicated pregnancies; these are then translated into more specific objectives that should be easier to audit or evaluate. Just a few of the possible objectives are listed.

Box 2.1: Aims and objectives of the 'Violet' Team for women with complicated pregnancies

Aims

For women with complications in pregnancy, birth and the puerperium:

1. To provide extra support throughout the childbearing period;
2. To improve continuity of care;
3. To ensure good communication between all relevant staff involved in a woman's care; and
4. To enhance midwifery skills.

Objectives *(could include)*

1. Violet Team aims to provide all the midwifery care for women regularly attending the special consultant antenatal clinic for the following reasons... *(specified)*.
2. Women referred to the team will be assessed at booking (or on referral) by a team midwife and an individual midwifery care plan agreed.
3. At antenatal visits to the hospital clinic, each woman will be cared for, wherever possible, by one of the two team members who have been assigned to her care.
4. Overall the woman should see not more than four different midwives in the course of her antenatal care.
5. Meetings between the Violet Team leader and relevant obstetricians should take place on a regular basis *(specified)*.
6. Midwives in the Violet Team will have the opportunity to attend *(specified)* study days and courses.
7. The Team's activities will be audited regularly. Responsibility for audit will rotate through all team members on a six monthly basis...........etc.

Formulating questions and deciding on the scale of the work

Preliminary work such as compiling a service description, formally writing down and getting agreement for the aims and objectives of the service and identifying issues which will be important to the evaluation, should all help in identifying the evaluation questions. A literature review and contact with databases of ongoing research and audit will help you to find out if other people have been looking at similar issues (see Chapter 10). It can make a great deal of difference to talk through your ideas with other people involved in evaluation. Local research groups and national initiatives, like the Changing Childbirth Team, can be useful for making contact.

If you are introducing an entirely new service, then you almost certainly should be undertaking some form of evaluation. The issue then is a question of the scale of the evaluation. Chapter 4 gives a number of examples of fairly large scale, more comprehensive evaluations, where many aspects of the services (health outcomes for women and babies, user views, staff views and costs) were investigated. Evaluations like these should be considered if your new service is a major departure from the way in which maternity care has been conventionally organized. On the other hand local implementation of schemes which have been tried and tested elsewhere should not require elaborate evaluation. This is a stage where it can be very useful to get help from experienced researchers.

Knowing when you need help

However keen you may be to undertake an evaluation yourself you may need to get help with it. Possible reasons for requiring assistance with an evaluation include:

- The need for the evaluation to be seen to be independent and objective
- Lack of time
- Lack of expertise
- An elaborate evaluation which will require a range of expertise.

It is a good idea to seek advice and comment when planning an evaluation: you don't have to take it but it's better to be aware of potential problems with it, and possible criticisms of it, before you start. Chapter 10 provides further guidance on the practical steps required when planning an evaluation and discusses how to go about getting expert help.

Thinking it through

This book should help you to judge when you need help and each chapter should help you to choose the most appropriate approach to your evaluation. However, before going ahead with an evaluation, it is important to stop and check whether you really want to proceed. Part of this involves thinking through exactly what will be involved and the possible consequences. Here are some questions that should be considered:

- Are you sure you have all the resources necessary to see the evaluation through to the end?
- What will you do if the evaluation shows that your way of organizing care is not working well?
- If the evaluation shows that your way of organizing care is working well, are those in your Trust, who are ultimately responsible for services, likely to be convinced by your findings? If the answer is no, is there another way of undertaking the evaluation the results of which they might find more convincing?

Further reading

There is a good discussion of the process of deciding on research questions in: Crombie, I.K., Davies, H.T.O. (1996). *Research in Health Care*. Chichester: Wiley.

There are also several references at the end of Chapter 10 to books which could help with this stage of a project.

CHAPTER THREE

Methods of Evaluation

Jo Garcia and Rona Campbell

In the first chapter *evaluation* was defined as attempting to find out if something was 'of value', if it worked as intended. This was contrasted with *research*, the aim of which was to generate new knowledge. *Audit*, it was suggested, was a form of evaluation, in that it was concerned with assessing if what should be happening, as determined by pre-set objectives or current knowledge, was actually happening. These activities, evaluation, audit and research, while different in their aims, can all use the same range of research methods and techniques.

Which methods are suitable to answer questions about the organization of maternity care? There is no single correct way of classifying the various types of methods in health services research. Different professions and disciplines approach this in different ways. At the end of this chapter there are suggestions of useful general books and articles that deal with a range of research approaches and techniques. We have adopted a different way to set out the various methods that may be suitable. Having suggested in the two preceding chapters that there are general goals which the maternity services should be trying to meet, and suggested some specific questions for each goal, we now discuss the methods that can be used to answer these questions.

Methods for addressing questions of safety and effectiveness

There are a variety of methods which might be used for addressing questions of safety and effectiveness including:

- Randomized controlled trials;
- Non-randomized comparisons;
- Studies of trends over time;
- Audits of agreed standards; and
- Staffing and workload models.

Randomized controlled trials are generally the first option to consider (see Boxes 3.1 and 3.2 for more detail on this method). Well designed trials give the least biased answers to questions about cause and effect and some trials of organizational aspects of maternity care have been done (e.g. Flint and Poulengeris, 1987; Elbourne, et al., 1987; MacVicar et al., 1993; Sikorski et al., 1996; Hundley et al., 1994; Turnbull et al.,

1995; Tucker et al., 1996). In maternity care, a useful introduction to the rationale for randomized controlled trials and a summary of findings in many areas is *A Guide to Effective Care in Pregnancy and Childbirth* (Enkin et al., 1995).

Box 3.1: Randomized controlled trials and non randomized comparisons

Randomized controlled trials (RCTs)

RCTs are based on the experimental format used in the physical and natural sciences. In health research RCTs are most commonly used to establish whether one treatment or intervention (e.g. indomethacin to stop pre-term labour) is more or less effective than another, but this method can also be used to test the effectiveness of different ways of organizing care (e.g. midwife or consultant led care for women with uncomplicated pregnancies). In maternity care the subjects are usually the women receiving the care but they could also be the care providers.

In a simple RCT, subjects are randomly allocated into experimental (new treatment) and control (no or existing treatment) groups. Each subject has exactly the same chance of being in the experimental or control group, thereby ensuring that there are no systematic differences in the characteristics of those in the two groups. Any differences in outcome observed between the two groups can then be attributed to the different 'treatments' which the two groups received.

Non randomized comparisons

These designs are similar to RCTs but subjects are not randomized into groups. In evaluations of the organization of care, comparisons are often made between one maternity unit or trust into which a new form of care organization has been introduced and another where the conventional way of providing care is still in operation. The evaluation of One-to-One midwifery in Queen Charlotte's Hospital in London has used this approach (McCourt and Page, 1996).

Comparisons of outcomes for women and babies cared for under a new form of care with those who were cared for under the previous system of organizing care (control) within the same maternity unit or trust, the so called 'before and after trial' is another example of a non randomized study design.

The absence of randomization means that the groups may not be alike. Thus, any differences in outcome may be due to pre-existing differences between the two groups, rather than the result of the alternative ways in which care was organized.

Numbers required

Calculations need to be made prior to undertaking a trial to estimate how many subjects will be required in order to have a reasonable likelihood of detecting differences between the experimental and control groups.

In some cases, though, it is not possible to do a trial. It may be that there is concern about a rare but serious outcome of care. To take this to extremes, consider the possibility that a new way of organizing care is putting mothers' or babies' lives at risk.

Death is a rare outcome in maternity care in this country. It would be almost impossible to do a trial to judge whether, say, a particular policy for referral to an obstetrician was more likely to lead to perinatal deaths than traditional care because so many women would need to be randomized. This dilemma is well illustrated in the debate about place of birth (Campbell and Macfarlane, 1994), where evidence about trends in mortality has been used to try to argue for and against the option of birth outside consultant obstetric units. It is usually less difficult to design trials that look at more common outcomes like rates of intervention in labour, breastfeeding success or admission to neonatal intensive care. Even for these outcomes, though, the numbers of women that we need to include in a study can be very large.

Box 3.2: Common misunderstandings about controlled trials

- Random allocation is the same as random sampling
  Random allocation means that subjects are allocated to groups in such a way that each has the same chance of being allocated to any group. Random sampling is quite different in that subjects are selected (sampled) from a group (population) in such a way that each has the same chance of being chosen.

- Should have same number of cases in treatment and control group
  A common method of randomly allocating subjects to experimental and control groups is to have opaque envelopes inside which there is a slip of paper with *experiment* or *control* written on it. When a subject has agreed to participate in a trial, they or a carer draws an envelop from a large box. The number of envelopes with either *experiment* or *control* slips should exceed the number of subjects required for the trial. If not, bias could creep in because, towards the end of the trial, the person drawing the envelope may be able to deduce what's inside the envelope if they know all the 'experimental' slips have already been allocated. Thus, it is unlikely that experimental and control groups will have exactly the same numbers in each group and you should be suspicious of any trial in which this appears to be the case. (There are more complex restricted randomization procedures which can be employed to ensure numbers in the treatment groups are approximately equal.)

- Experiments are unethical because they deny treatment to one group
  Trials of different methods of organizing care do not involve denying anyone care. Subjects may have a preference for one form of care and may be disappointed if not randomly allocated to this, but informed consent is an essential prerequisite before any patient is recruited to a trial. Not to obtain this would be unethical.

  Controlled trials are the only way of establishing cause and effect, therefore all evaluations of the organization of maternity care should be undertaken by means of a randomized trial. Randomized trials are the only way of unequivocally establishing cause and effect relationships, but there are other *what* and *why* questions in evaluations which can not readily be answered by randomized trials.

Some studies use a comparative approach, but without randomization. So, for example, women cared for by midwives newly organized into teams or group practices may be compared with other women using the same hospital but cared for in the usual way. Care may also be compared with that received by women in the same place before the changes took place (often called 'before and after' study or study with historical controls). There are many evaluations using these types of approaches (see for example Watson, 1990; McCourt and Page, 1996). It has the advantage of 'naturalness' because care givers do not have to alter what they are doing for the sake of the research, but the disadvantage is that interpretation is difficult because the women being compared may differ in known and unknown ways. These issues are taken up in more detail in Chapter 4.

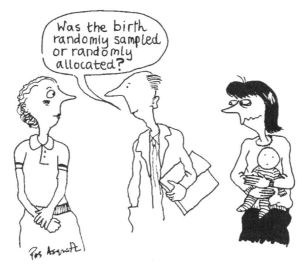

There are other non-experimental ways of looking at the safety and effectiveness of different patterns of care. They give an indication of whether care is likely to be safe and effective. By using audit approaches we can see if care measures are up to agreed standards. Standards can be set on the basis of evidence – for example, if, based on reliable evidence, the policy is that certain categories of women in pre-term labour should be given corticosteroids antenatally to improve their babies' lung maturity, then audit can tell us if this is being done. Other safety standards can be based on partial evidence with the addition of experience and common sense. By reviewing care records, we can find out if the tests and treatments given to women with an inherited condition like thalassaemia are in line with the current policies. We can look at women cared for in a new way to see if some problems like pre-eclampsia or malpresentation are being adequately identified. These audits of clinical standards are time consuming to do, but can provide useful information.

Another approach to safety is to look at the number, qualifications and experience of staff available to provide care at different times. This may be linked to the specific needs of the women and babies passing through that maternity unit. Planned and achieved staffing can then be compared, using hypothetical modelling approaches, with the levels recommended on the basis of various models (Ball and Washbrook, 1996). Linked to this are issues about appropriate referral to specialists and super-specialists. Which categories of women should see an obstetrician antenatally? Should the GP or midwife have access to ultrasound without referral to an obstetrician? Should women with heart disease or diabetes be referred to a specialist obstetrician or physician? Overall, the issue of safety is a difficult one to resolve. Those in favour of a new model of care are often challenged to show that it is as safe as the old way of working. In practice this is very difficult to do because maternal and infant deaths are now so rare that statistically significant differences will only be detected if very large numbers are studied. National data on maternity care outcomes and the national confidential enquiries into maternal deaths and the stillbirths and deaths in infancy (CESDI) are crucial for monitoring the overall safety and quality of the services.

In general, the methods that are used to answer questions about safety and effectiveness have been developed within a branch of health research known as epidemiology. This is concerned with trying to understand disease processes and their causes by looking at the pattern of disease within populations. These methods therefore tend to rely on large numbers and statistical analysis. On the other hand, smaller scale, more descriptive studies can raise questions about safety which can then be explored in other ways. At the end of this chapter there is advice about general books and articles which may be helpful if you want to look at the epidemiological and statistical background to your evaluation.

Methods for assessing what women and their families think of maternity service

If care is to be properly evaluated, we need to have reliable ways to find out about women's views and experiences. There are lots of different approaches to getting women's views and these are described in more detail in Chapter 5. Postal surveys have been the method used most often, but interviews, focus group discussions and observation of care are also important. There has been little work so far on the advantages and disadvantages of the different methods. Work on the experiences of those who use the health services can be large scale and quantitative or much more descriptive. Some randomized controlled trials include an assessment of women's views of care. The Know-your-midwife trial, for example, studied the impact of care from a small team of midwives on women's physical and emotional well-being (Flint and Poulengeris, 1987). Other studies use very small samples to understand an area in depth.

Survey methods (see Box 3.3) are very widely used, but there are some common misunderstandings about them (see Box 3.4) and they are often very badly executed. Surveys, particularly those done by postal questionnaire, can appear deceptively simple and cheap to the uninitiated. A form is designed with a series of questions, these are sent out, the respondents do the bulk of the work by filling the questionnaire in, the answers are fed into a computer package which aggregates all the responses and 'hey presto' your evaluation is done. The reality is that designing a good questionnaire, obtaining a high level of response from a representative sample and compiling and analysing the data well requires considerable skill. If you are designing a questionnaire from scratch you can expect to have to produce up to ten drafts and to pilot it (i.e. test it out in a limited way) several times before it will be ready for use. Several of the texts recommended at the end of this chapter, in particular that by de Vaus (1993), should help to ensure that any survey you undertake is of a high quality.

Box 3.3: Survey methods

- Surveys are used to obtain a representative picture of what is happening or what people think. Rather than survey an entire group, surveys are usually undertaken on a random sample of the total group or population. Statistical theory is then used to make generalizations from the sample survey information to the population as a whole. Such generalizations can only be undertaken if random sampling methods have been used.

- Survey research has almost become synonymous with questionnaires. Although this is undoubtedly the most common method of data collection, data in a survey can also be collected through a variety of means including observation or a semi-structured interview. The distinguishing characteristic is that the same pieces of information (variables) have to be collected about every individual in the survey.

- Surveys tend to be used simply to describe people's views or document what is happening, but one or more pieces of information from a survey can be examined simultaneously. For example, some surveys of user satisfaction have found that women having their babies at home have enjoyed the birth more than when they gave birth in hospital (Campbell and Macfarlane, 1994). One might conclude that this means that having a home birth produces greater satisfaction i.e. that there is a cause and effect relationship. This is incorrect, however. Surveys indicate associations but only randomized trials can provide concrete evidence of cause and effect.

- As with randomized trials it is important to calculate how large the sample for your survey needs to be in order to be able to make reasonable generalizations to the population as a whole.

Box 3.4: Common misunderstandings about survey methods

- You can get a survey to demonstrate whatever you want. The 'spoof' questions overleaf would seem to prove the point. What they actually illustrate, however, is that any series of biased or loaded questions will produce biased answers.

- The larger the size of the sample in relation to the total population, the more representative it is. While intuitively this might seem to be the case, statistical theory has it otherwise. It is the absolute, rather than the relative size of the sample that matters. The larger the absolute size of the sample, the smaller the sampling error, that is, the error which is incurred because you have not included every member of the population.

- Surveys are always undertaken with individual people as the unit of enquiry. Although most surveys are undertaken using individual respondents as the 'survey' unit there is no reason why the survey unit could not be a collectivity, such as a general practice or a maternity unit or a trust.

Place of Birth – It's your choice!

Questionnaires can sometimes be biased – the questions may have been designed to get a particular answer. Imagine a political battle over place of birth and some of the questions that women could be asked. Looking at the two sets of questions below, it's easy to see how the answer to the final question on place of birth might be influenced by the biased or loaded nature of the preceding questions.

Set One

How important is it to you to give birth in the safety of a hospital labour ward, with specialist doctors on the spot?

　　Very important　　　　　　Fairly important　　　　　　Not important

To what extent do you agree that safety should be the overriding consideration in choice of place of birth?

　　Strongly agree　　Agree　　No view　　Disagree　　Strongly disagree

How important is it to you that you have hospital doctors and midwives to look after and advise you in the first few days after the baby is born?

　　Very important　　　　　　Fairly important　　　　　　Not important

Where would you like to give birth to your next baby?

　　In hospital　　　　　　At home　　　　　　Some other place

Set Two

The peaceful and private environment of the woman's own home is best for baby and mother.

　　Strongly agree　　Agree　　No view　　Disagree　　Strongly disagree

How important is it to you to avoid the risks of infection and unnecessary intervention in a hospital labour ward?

　　Very important　　　　　　Fairly important　　　　　　Not important

How important is it to you to have your own GP and community midwife to visit you at home and your family to look after you in the first few days after the baby is born?

　　Very important　　　　　　Fairly important　　　　　　Not important

Where would you like to give birth to your next baby?

　　In hospital　　　　　　At home　　　　　　Some other place

These questions were made up to illustrate a point and there are other problems with them besides the fact that they are hopelessly biased. Unfortunately, there are plenty of real examples of biased questionnaires and opinion polls. It may be easy to avoid crude bias but it is not easy to design good, clear, unbiased and unambiguous questions. Useful books on questionnaire design and other aspects of survey methods are listed at the end of this chapter.

Research about the views of service users also draws upon approaches under the broad heading of 'qualitative' research (see Boxes 3.5 and 3.6). A number of approaches can be listed under this heading. One such approach, which is very relevant to evaluation of the organization of maternity services, is ethnography. It is generally understood to involve the researcher(s) 'participating, overtly or covertly, in people's daily lives for an extended period of time, watching what happens, listening to what is said, asking questions – in fact collecting whatever data are available to throw light on the issues that are the focus of the research' (Hammersley and Atkinson, 1995). Field work is another term which in practice means much the same thing. There are other more specialized approaches or methods such as oral history (Leap and Hunter, 1993) or discourse analysis which only have a very limited role in the evaluation of the organization of maternity care and are therefore not discussed further in this book.

Qualitative methods often aim to see things through the eyes of those being studied. In the case of maternity services, this could mean both those providing and those receiving care. Thus, qualitative methods are useful when investigating women's views and knowledge of the services available to them. They are also useful in looking at issues of sustainability, in particular how maternity staff feel about changes to the organization of care (see Chapter 6). Qualitative methods are descriptive and exploratory. They are thus particularly useful when trying to answer 'why' type questions. They have their origins in the social sciences, unlike randomized and non randomized trials or survey research, whose origins lie in the physical sciences. Qualitative methods are therefore informed by a quite different philosophical basis and are not concerned with cause and effect but with understanding. Because in qualitative research the researcher is the research instrument, good qualitative researchers think very carefully about the effect that they might be having on those they are studying (the technical name given to this is reactivity). They pay particular attention to what effects their own thoughts, biases and feelings may have on the way they collect their data and interpret it. The qualitative researcher often records these thoughts in a separate 'reflexive account'. Sheila Hunt's (1995) ethnographic study of what happens in a labour ward entitled *The Social Meaning of Midwifery* provides an excellent example of good ethnography by a reflexive researcher.

Methods of evaluating whether particular ways of organizing maternity care are sustainable

This is primarily investigated by economic analyses which are covered in Chapter 7. Human resources are part of the economic picture but there need to be other ways of looking at the impact of changes in care on the staff involved. At a national level it may be useful to use professional registers to see who is entering and leaving the professions and to inform discussions on training, recruitment and retention. Surveys of staff can provide important information both nationally and locally about the aspirations and views of those providing the care. At a local level there are interesting studies that look in depth at the way that staff work together, and how they react to change. These issues are discussed in more detail in Chapter 6 and a qualitative study that deals with the use of registrar and consultant grades in obstetrics is discussed as one of the examples in Chapter 4.

Box 3.5: Characteristics of qualitative methods

Looking at things from the point of view of those being studied

This can be achieved by observation (either as a participant or a non participant in the activity being studied) or by in depth interviewing where the questions asked are open ended.

Trying to understand

The role of the researcher in qualitative work is to try and understand what is really going on, rather than what is assumed to be happening. For example, in her study of waiting lists, Catherine Pope found that lists were not orderly queues of people with those who had been in the queue longest or those in the greatest need of treatment being dealt with first (Pope, 1993). By observing what actually happened in the offices where appointments for treatment were made, she found that waiting lists were in fact used like a pool of patients which clinicians drew on. Thus, someone might be selected for treatment because the clinician knew them or found them to be a particularly interesting case rather than take whoever was next in line.

Holism, naturalism and process

Qualitative research tends to focus on the process by which things happen as much as on their outcome. To do this, the researcher has to go where the people are and observe or talk to them in their own 'natural' surroundings. In the case of maternity service users, this will probably either mean their home or the institutional settings in which care is given. Qualitative research also tends to take a holistic view of what is happening and look at it from every angle rather than focusing on selected aspects. To do this qualitative researchers often write very detailed descriptions and keep a journal of how the research is progressing. It also may mean using a number of different methods and perhaps involving more than one researcher. Most of all holism means recognizing that for individuals there can be many realities and that individuals may hold contradictory ideas and views.

Flexibility

In seeking to achieve objectivity quantitative research follows very precise formats. Qualitative research is conducted in a much less rigid way. A quantitative piece of research usually begins with a formal hypothesis which is tested during the course of the research, for example, 'There is no difference in the continuity of care provided by midwives, whether they are organized into teams or each manage their own caseload'. In qualitative research the initial question may simply be the very general one, 'What constitutes continuity of care and how is it understood by those who provide and receive care?'. Flexibility also means being prepared to change your whole approach once the research is underway if you find it isn't working.

> **Box 3.6:** Common misunderstandings about qualitative methods
>
> - Because it's flexible, it's easy to do.
>   People who are uncomfortable with numerical or highly structured research methods sometimes opt for qualitative research because they think it will be easier. Although qualitative research isn't governed by the same kinds of formal rules which frame survey or experimental research, the choice of method and technique in qualitative work has to be justified and the wrong choice will result in failure just as it would in quantitative work.
>
> - It is less time consuming than quantitative work.
>   Observing or interviewing can be very time consuming and exhausting. It can take from four to six hours, sometimes even longer, to transcribe one hour of an interview tape. Reading and rereading transcripts and classifying and coding sections of text as part of the analysis is also very time consuming.
>
> - It doesn't prove anything.
>   Qualitative research isn't about proving, it is about understanding. Thus, one may be able to demonstrate with an experimental approach that a particular way of organizing care did not produce the desired outcome but a qualitative approach would help to identify why the scheme failed.

Methods for assessing efficiency

Audits of care and studies of working patterns provide information about efficiency. Studies could cover the availability of records and test results, the communication between hospital and community staff or the time spent travelling in relation to visit times. Studies of computerized information systems have looked at the quality of data stored and at ease of access and the possibility of making changes in the data items collected. Data from surveys of women might also indicate problems with efficiency, for example, where appointments were cancelled at short notice, or notes were missing.

Methods of evaluating accessibility and equity in the organization of maternity care

The types of studies that are useful to provide evidence about equity and accessibility include surveys and the use of routinely collected data. Good data are needed to compare the care that women get in different settings and to explore the extent that care is relevant to what is needed. Questions of equity and accessibility can be addressed using classic epidemiological methods – that is by monitoring trends and studying the geographical and social distribution of relevant characteristics. For example, one might wish to monitor rates of teenage pregnancy in geographically defined areas and then examine whether the maternity care facilities in each of the areas was providing the kind of care that was sensitive to the needs of young mothers. Local studies of maternity care carried out by purchasers have used surveys of women and audits to explore differences in the services available to resident women at different trusts serving the population, and investigated care for groups with particular needs like women from minority ethnic groups (e.g. Hemingway et al., 1994). Such studies may be hampered though by small numbers; regional or national studies may be better for some topics. Local studies may also be able to compare their findings with national data. Help with work of this kind is most likely to come from local academic departments of public health, or from public health doctors.

Box 3.7: Reliability and validity

Whatever the question you are intending to answer, it is important to consider whether the approach you take is likely to yield accurate answers. There are two rather abstract components to accuracy in a research context:

- **Reliability:** that is whether the measurement or observation you are making is dependable so that if you were to make it repeatedly you would get the same thing each time.

- **Validity:** that is whether what you are measuring or observing is sound or true. In other words is it what you intended to measure?

Issues of reliability and validity are important in both qualitative and quantitative research but are dealt with rather differently. The text books on the different methods recommended under 'further reading' have sections dealing with these issues.

Having described the various approaches that can be taken, it should be clear that to use any one demands rigor and requires skill. The method or methods should always be chosen on the basis that they are appropriate to the question(s) posed in the evaluation.

References

Ball, J., Washbrook, M. (1996). *Birthrate Plus*. Hale, Cheshire: Books for Midwives Press.

Campbell, R., Macfarlane, A. (1994). *Where to Be Born?* Second Edition. Oxford: National Perinatal Epidemiology Unit.

Elbourne, D., Richardson, M., Chalmers, I., Waterhouse, I., Holt, E. (1987). 'The Newbury maternity care study: a randomised controlled trial to assess a policy of women holding their own obstetric records'. *Br J Obs & Gynaecol*, Vol. 94, pp. 612–619.

Enkin, M., Keirse, M.J.C.N., Renfrew, M., Neilson, J. (1995). *A Guide to Effective Care in Pregnancy and Childbirth*. Oxford: Oxford University Press.

Flint, C., Poulengeris, P. (1987). *The 'Know your Midwife' Report*. 49 Peckarmans Wood, London SE26 6RZ.

Hemingway, H., Saunders, D., Parsons, L. (1994). *Women's Experiences of Maternity Services in East London: An Evaluation*. London: East London and City Health Authority.

Hundley, V., Cruickshank, F., Lang, G. et al. (1994). 'Midwife managed delivery unit: a randomised controlled comparison with consultant led care'. *BMJ*, Vol. 309, pp. 1400–1404.

Hunt, S., Symonds, A. (1995). *The Social Meaning of Midwifery*. London: Macmillan.

Leap, N., Hunter, B. (1993). *The Midwife's Tale: An Oral History from Handywoman to Professional Midwife*. London: Scarlet Press.

MacVicar, J., Dobbie, G., Owen-Johnstone, L. et al. (1993). 'Simulated home delivery in hospital: a randomised controlled trial'. *British Journal of Obstetrics and Gynaecology*, Vol. 100, pp. 316–23.

McCourt, C., Page, L. (Eds.) (1996). *Report on the Evaluation of One to One Midwifery Practice*. London: The Hammersmith Hospital NHS Trust & Thames Valley University.

Pope, C. (1993). 'Trouble in store: some thoughts on the management of waiting lists'. *Sociology of Health and Illness*, Vol. 13, pp. 193–212.

Sikorski, J., Wilson, J., Clement, S. et al. (1996). 'A randomized trial comparing two schedules of antenatal visits: the antenatal care project'. *BMJ*, Vol. 312, pp. 546–53.

Tucker, J.S., Hall, M.H., Howie, P.W. et al. (1996). 'Should obstetricians see women with normal pregnancies? A multicentre randomised controlled trial of routine antenatal care by general practitioners and midwives compared with shared care lead by obstetricians'. *BMJ*, Vol. 312, pp. 554–59.

Turnbull, D., Reid, M., McGinley, M., Sheilds, N.R. (1995). 'Changes in midwives' attitudes to their professional role following the implementation of the midwifery development unit'. *Midwifery*, Vol. 11, pp. 110–119.

Watson, P. (1990). *Report on the Kidlington Team Midwifery Scheme*. Oxford: Institute of Nursing.

Further reading

Survey methods

de Vaus, D. (1993). *Surveys in Social Research*. London: UCL Press.

Cartwright, A. (1983). *Health Surveys in Practice and in Potential: A Critical Review of their Scope and Methods*. London: King's Fund.

Oppenheim, A.N. (1992). *Questionnaire Design, Interviewing and Attitude Measurement*. London: Pinter Publishers. (New Edition).

Experimental methods

Pocock, S. (1983). *Clinical Trials: A Practical Approach*. Chichester: John Wiley.

Chalmers, I., Enkin, M., Keirse, M. ((1989). *Effective Care in Pregnancy and Childbirth*. Oxford: Oxford University Press.

Clegg, F. (1982). *Simple Statistics*. Cambridge: Cambridge University Press.

Qualitative methods

Mays, N., Pope, C. (1996). *Qualitative Research in Health Care*. London: British Medical Journal Publishing Group.

Hammersley, M., Atkinson, P. (1995). *Ethnography: Principles in Practice*. Second edition. London: Routledge.

Morse, J.M. (1992). *Qualitative Health Research*. London: Sage.

Hunt, S., Symonds, A. (1995). *The Social Meaning of Midwifery*. Basingstoke: Macmillan.

Audit and quality assurance

Crombie, I.K., Davies, H.T.O., Abraham, S.C.S., Florey, C.V. (1993). *The Audit Handbook*. Chichester: John Wiley.

Downe, S. (1994). 'Maternity audit in practice'. *British Journal of Midwifery*, Vol. 2, pp. 77–82.

Ball, J., Hughes, D. (1993). 'Quality assurance in maternity care'. In: Bennett, V.L., Brown, L.K. (Eds). *Myles Textbook for Midwives*. 12th Edition. Edinburgh: Churchill Livingstone.

Baker, R. (1988). *Practice Assessment and Quality Care*. London: Royal College of General Practitioners.

General texts

Crombie, I.K., Davies, H.T.O. (1996). *Research in Health Care*. Chichester: Wiley.
This is a very useful general text, with a lot of good examples and interesting references.

Oakley, A. (1992). *Social Support and Motherhood*. Oxford: Basil Blackwell.
This account of a research project addressed many issues about the choice of methods and about some of the practical aspects of getting funding and carrying out a study

Brown, S., Lumley, J., Small, R., Astbury, J. (1994). *Missing Voices: The Experience of Motherhood*. Oxford: Oxford University Press.
This is another report of a research project that covers a range of methodological issues in a clear and useful way.

Hilton, A. (1987). *The Ethnographic Perspective*. Research Awareness Module 7. London: South Bank Polytechnic, Distance Learning Centre.
Rodgers, J. (1988). *The Survey Perspective*. Research Awareness Module 8. London: South Bank Polytechnic, Distance Learning Centre.
Clark, E. (1988). *The Experimental Perspective*. Research Awareness Module 9. London: South Bank Polytechnic, Distance Learning Centre.
Clark, E., Renfrew, M. (1992). 'Research awareness and the midwife'. *Midwifery Update*. Module 9. London: South Bank Polytechnic, Distance Learning Centre.

These excellent publications may be available in academic and health service libraries. They cannot be bought in bookshops but, with the exception of Clark and Renfrew (1992) which is out of print, all are available from T.B.C. Distribution, South Lodge, Gravesend Road, Routeham, Kent TN15 7JJ. Tel: 01732 824700. They are course materials from distance learning packages. They are thus designed to provide the reader with knowledge of particular research methods and enable them to acquire certain research skills.

CHAPTER FOUR

Evaluating the Organization of Maternity Care from a Number of Perspectives

Rona Campbell

'Better understanding of the effects of different models of care on service users would be useful, including qualitative research on users views and perspectives. A further important strand of work is the effects on service providers, including descriptive work on existing patterns of care and evaluations of new configurations of services and models of care... Above all, there is a need to demonstrate that major changes in service provision do not have adverse side effects on the safety of mothers and their offspring.' (Department of Health, 1995)

This chapter looks at the ways in which it is possible to conduct more comprehensive evaluations, involving a variety of outcome measures and including attempts to assess the safety and effectiveness of different ways of organizing maternity care. Such evaluations tend to be larger in scale than many described to date in this book and could involve a number of centres. As a result they require detailed planning and considerable expertise in research methods. They are also costly both in financial and personnel terms. Subsequent chapters focus on the evaluation of specific types of outcome, for example, user satisfaction or costs.

The purpose of this chapter is to illustrate, using real examples, the range of approaches that can be taken. The studies cited have been chosen because their findings were important and illuminating. Although all are good they should not to be regarded as ideal models. Each had minor difficulties, some of which have been pointed out by the authors, and others by correspondents to the journals in which the findings were published.

Randomized trial

This approach, which is regarded by many as the only one capable of providing unequivocal evidence that one system of care is more effective than another, is increasingly being used in evaluations of the organization of maternity care. One such study was that undertaken in Aberdeen to compare a new midwifery managed delivery unit with consultant led care. Midwifery led units are a relatively new form of care and the evaluation of the Aberdeen Unit was only the second to have been published. It is important because it attempted to evaluate how safe, effective, acceptable and efficient this form of care was in comparison to delivery in a labour ward (Hundley et al., 1994).

The stated objective of the study was to 'examine whether intrapartum care and delivery of low risk women in a midwife managed delivery unit differs from that in a consultant led ward'. To assess this, 2844 women who met booking criteria for delivery in general practitioner units in the locality were randomized at booking to delivery in the midwife managed unit or the labour ward. For every one woman randomized to the labour ward, two were randomized for delivery in the midwife managed unit. Due to the fact that women who developed complications during pregnancy and labour were transferred to consultant led care, the disproportionate allocation to the midwives unit ensured that it retained a viable workload during the trial.

Box 4.1: Outcome measures for the Aberdeen trial

- Maternal and infant mortality
- Maternal and infant morbidity
- Complication rates
- Intervention rates
- Users experiences and satisfaction
- Midwives experiences and satisfaction
- Costs of care

The rarity of stillbirth, neonatal death or life threatening morbidity in mother or baby, makes assessing the relative safety of different models of care in single trials using these outcome measures very difficult. Thus, most recent trials have focused on proxy measures of more serious morbidity. These include such indicators as low Apgar scores and resuscitation rates in neonates, non life threatening (though distressing) morbidity such as tearing or episiotomy in women, intervention rates and process measures such as transfer rates and type of staff undertaking the delivery. The trial in Aberdeen went further than this and a wide range of outcome measures were recorded (Box 4.1). This necessitated collecting data from a number of sources during the trial (Box 4 2).

Box 4.2: Data collection for the Aberdeen trial

- Questionnaire completed by midwife in charge of delivery
- Questionnaire completed by mother after discharge
- Interview with random sample of study population
- Information collected from:
  Scottish Morbidity Register (SMR2)
  Aberdeen Maternity and Neonatal Databank
  Case note review

Assessing safety

The data from the trial were analysed according to what is known as the 'intention to treat' principle (Newell, 1992). This meant that the data analysis was based on the groups to which women were originally randomized, rather than the places in which they actually gave birth. As the randomization took place at booking, the trial was in effect evaluating all the care from then on and not, as the authors of the study have suggested, just the care around the time of birth (Smith, 1995).

The first results of the trial were published in the *British Medical Journal* (BMJ) and the authors concluded that the study 'confirms that midwife managed care is as safe as standard consultant led care'. The findings showed that there were no statistically significant difference in maternal and neonatal mortality or morbidity. It was, however, pointed out in letters published subsequently in the BMJ, that the trial was too small to have had the statistical power to detect differences in mortality or in life threatening forms of morbidity, and that the trial could not have answered questions about safety (Brocklehurst et al., 1995). The authors had, in fact, indicated that they were aware of this problem and had therefore focused on morbidity 'as the principal measure of outcome'. A similar study involving 814 women, conducted in Australia, which compared the outcomes for mothers and babies of care provided by midwives working in a team with that provided routinely by a variety of doctors and midwives, also acknowledged the problem of having a trial with sufficiently large numbers of women in it to detect statistically significant differences in mortality or life threatening morbidity. They noted that 'Continuity of care provided by a small team of midwives resulted in a more satisfying birth experience at less cost than routine care and fewer adverse maternal and neonatal outcomes. Although a much larger study would be required to provide adequate power to detect rare outcomes, our study found that continuity of care by a midwife team was as safe as routine care' (Rowley et al., 1995).

As these examples show, definitions of what constitutes safety can vary. They also indicate that if safety is measured in terms of death or the presence of life threatening morbidity, then a single trial is rarely sufficient to establish the safety of a new way of delivering maternity care. It is only when the results of a number of trials are aggregated, using a procedure known as meta-analysis, or when all the evidence has been systematically reviewed, that a particular practice, procedure or method of organizing care can be deemed safe and effective. Pooling results, however, is not always straight forward. Models of maternity care may be delivered in different settings, to differing groups of women, by staff whose levels of knowledge and skill may vary in ways which could affect the outcomes of the deliveries.

The views of midwives

The questionnaire, completed shortly after the delivery of a women in the trial by the midwife in charge, contained questions about continuity of care and the qualifications and experience of the staff giving care. There was also a section on which the midwife could record her level of satisfaction on a scale from 0 to 10 (0 indicating 'Throughout unsatisfactory. Nothing good to be said about it' and 10 'An absolutely wonderful experience that could not have been better') and her overall impression of the delivery. Other clinical data relating to the labour and delivery were also recorded on this questionnaire. Booking for delivery in the midwife led unit was found to be associated with greater continuity of care during labour and after. There was a statistically significant but small difference in midwives' overall levels of satisfaction, with satisfaction being greater among midwives working in the midwife led unit. Nevertheless, the best predictors of midwife satisfaction were not the kind of booking or where the birth took place but the degree of midwife autonomy and continuity of carer (Hundley, 1995a).

In this trial midwifery staff rotated through the delivery suite according to clinical need and therefore midwives may have treated women in both groups. Nevertheless, one of the reasons for the greater continuity of carer achieved in the midwife led unit may have been that because the more experienced midwifery staff spent longer working in it, they did not need to seek medical assistance with certain procedures. The existence of this possible source of bias highlights one of the key difficulties in a trial of this nature. While randomization of women to the two different forms of care excludes one source of bias, it is more difficult to eliminate possible biases in the groups of staff providing the care in the different settings. Randomizing staff is a possible but often impractical solution to this.

Another difficulty in interpreting the results from this study was that only one very simple indicator of midwife satisfaction was used and the authors acknowledged that a more detailed instrument might have produced more conclusive results.

Costs of introducing the midwife led unit

After the completion of the trial an economic evaluation was undertaken to assess the additional cost (or saving) per woman of introducing the midwifery led unit. Data from the trial indicating resource use was employed but supplementary information on costs had to be derived from a variety of sources including hospital statistics, administrative data on costs of different services, theatre records and an ad hoc questionnaire (Hundley, 1995b).

The costs measured in the evaluation, and the total cost per woman of introducing midwife led care according to each cost category, are indicated in Box 4.3. The largest contribution to the total cost per women delivered was the midwifery staff costs which amounted to the equivalent of employing three extra grade F midwives and promoting seven midwives from E to F grades. Although the introduction of the midwifery unit resulted in an increase in the grade and numbers of midwives beyond what would have been required on a labour ward, as 46 per cent of women booked for the midwifery unit actually delivered there without medical assistance, no mention is made of a possible cost saving because consultant cover was no longer required. Such cover might have been deemed necessary had these women been booked for delivery under a system of consultant led care.

Box 4.3: Costs measures in the Aberdeen trial

Staff costs

The costs of midwifery staff employed in the midwife led unit which were in addition to those required if women had been booked on the labour ward.

Staff time costed where there were statistically significant differences in intervention rates. Where differences were not statistically significant but there was likely to have been an impact on clinical practice and resource use (e.g. caesarean section, assisted vaginal delivery, general anaesthetic) such differences were costed.

Additional staff cost per woman of midwife led care: £44.69

Capital costs

Cost of converting a wing of the delivery suite into the midwife led unit
Cost of equipment used in midwife led unit
Cost of equipment required if midwife led unit became a labour ward

Capital cost saving per woman of midwife led care: £0.73

Consumables

Market values of consumables associated with statistically significant and clinically significant differences identified in the two arms of the trial

Consumable cost saving per woman of midwife led care: £3.25

Total cost per woman: £40.70

(Source: Hundley, 1995b)

Costing packages of health care is often an inexact science and assumptions and estimates have to be made. By varying systematically each assumption and estimate made in a series of scenarios, it is possible to test their effects on the overall costings. The technical name for this process is a sensitivity analysis. In the Aberdeen trial, a series of nine different scenarios were computed. These showed that the cost of introducing a new midwifery unit varied from an additional cost of £44.23 to a saving of £9.74.

It has often been assumed that adopting midwife led care will result in cost savings. The economic evaluation of the Aberdeen trial has highlighted that this is not necessarily so. It is important to recognize, however, that this economic evaluation was focused on the cost of *introducing* midwife led care not on a direct comparison of the costs of running consultant led and midwife led care.

Data on user satisfaction were collected as part of this evaluation but at the time of writing the analysis of these were still to be published.

Large scale, comprehensive evaluations such as that undertaken in Aberdeen are expensive. This one was funded by the Scottish Home and Health Department and cost £75, 000 over two years. In addition, six months of a health economist's time was required to complete the economic evaluation (Hundley, Personal communication).

Randomizing women to experimental and control groups should ensure that the characteristics of the women in both groups are the same. Thus, any differences in outcome observed between the two groups can be attributed to the different systems of care to which they were allocated. There are, however, situations where it is not feasible to undertake a randomized trial. Then a quasi experimental approach (i.e. non-randomized comparison) can be a useful alternative. This can take a number of forms including a natural experiment and a before and after design. Both of these approaches are discussed below.

Natural experiment

If a particular change or intervention has been introduced in one place and not in another, this can be viewed as the basis for natural experiment and comparisons can be made between the outcomes achieved in the two different places. A recent independent evaluation of team midwifery by the Institute of Public Health at the University of Cambridge contained elements in which comparisons were made within the framework of a natural experiment (Farquhar et al., 1996). Seven teams of community midwives, each with seven WTE midwives, provided antenatal, intrapartum and postnatal care to women in the district studied. A further 37 midwives (core staff) were hospital based.

While not comprehensive in the sense that it did not involve any costing or attempt to assess cost effectiveness, this evaluation was wide ranging in that it involved a case study, a postal survey of maternity care providers and users, the collection of process and outcome data and an audit of midwifery contacts. A brief description of each of these elements is given in Box 4.4.

Women receiving all their maternity care from team midwives in the district were included in the study group. These women either gave birth at home or in consultant obstetric units in hospitals within the district. Data gathered on and from these women were compared with data from three 'naturally occurring control groups':

1. Women who gave birth in a consultant unit within the district but were cared for antenatally and postnatally by community midwives from another district.
2. Women who gave birth either in a maternity unit near to but outside the district, or at home, and received their antenatal and postnatal care from a group of three midwives employed by a hospital within the district, but who did not work as a team.
3. Women who received their antenatal and postnatal care from one of the district midwifery teams but who delivered in a maternity unit outside the district.

Box 4.4: Methods used in an evaluation of midwifery teams

Case study

Unstructured interviews with key informants, together with a content analysis of relevant documentation such as minutes of meetings and protocols, were used to elucidate how and why team midwifery came into being. Developments in team midwifery which took place during the period of the evaluation were also tracked by these techniques.

Staff satisfaction survey

A literature search, and unstructured interviews with a small number of different staff providing maternity services, were used to identify the issues that should be covered in a postal questionnaire to be sent to all community and hospital midwives, general practitioners and health visitors in the district (Response rate: 83%).

User's survey

A questionnaire was developed based on one previously used at the obstetric unit at the hospital within the district. This was modified, to take account of issues identified in a literature review. For a six month period this questionnaire was sent, within a week of delivery, to all women delivering at the hospital obsteric unit within the district, or at home, and any women who had been cared for antenatally and postnatally by community midwives from the district but delivered in a maternity unit outside the district (Response rate: 88%).

An analysis of process and outcome data routinely collected by midwives

Routine data gathered by midwives at consultant obstetric units inside the district, on a range of outcome and process measures for women giving birth, were recorded on a form specifically designed for the evaluation. This was linked through the use of unique serial numbers to data from the user survey (95% completion rate).

An audit of midwife contacts

A form designed by the local clinical audit office was attached to the notes of all women given antenatal, intrapartum and postnatal care by a district midwifery team. On this form community midwives and women recorded the details of all antenatal contacts between the woman and the community midwives who cared for her. Through the use of serial numbers it was possible, on a case by case basis, to link these data to that from the user survey, and the process and outcome data (85 per cent completion rate obtained).

(Source: Farquhar et al., 1996)

The case study revealed that the move to team midwifery had largely been the result of the enthusiasm of one senior manager. Concern was expressed by some about the speed of implementation and whether the size of teams was correct.

The staff satisfaction survey, and in particular a part containing the Glasgow Midwifery Process Questionnaire, showed that there were 'significantly lower levels of professional satisfaction, client interaction and professional development scores for hospital midwives compared with community midwives but no differences in their professional support'. The majority of both hospital and community midwives thought team midwifery was a good idea in theory but 52 per cent of community midwives and 27 per cent of hospital midwives thought that quality of care had declined as a result of its introduction. Furthermore, only 45 per cent of community midwives and 19 per cent of hospital midwives thought the scheme was working well. General practitioners and health visitors expressed similar views.

Results from the user survey indicated that compared with women in the control groups, women in the study group had the lowest level of continuity of carer in the antenatal period. More than 75 per cent of women in the study group reported that they had seen 'a different midwife each time'. The second control group, who were the most likely to report only seeing 'just one or two midwives' and to report that they had formed a relationship with their midwives during the antenatal period, were, perhaps not surprisingly, the most satisfied with their care before labour. There were no differences between the study and control groups in levels of satisfaction with intrapartum or postnatal care.

Comparisons between the demographic characteristics of women in the study and control groups indicated some differences. Women in the study group tended to be younger, less well educated and living in council housing. This highlights one of the difficulties in interpreting findings from non randomized evaluations because it is possible, though in this case unlikely, that the differences between the types of women in the study and control groups explain the observed differences in satisfaction and continuity of care between the study and control groups. For example, it is possible that women in the control groups, who tended to be better educated, were more likely to identify with the midwives who cared for them. Conversely, women in the study groups may not have identified so closely with the midwives, and were therefore less likely to remember whether or not they had seen the same midwife. Thus, there might have been a tendency for women in the study group to under report continuity of care.

Analyses of the process and outcome data, however, indicated a high level of consistency between the information provided by midwives and details recorded by women themselves in the user survey. Overall, the process and outcome data illustrated that higher percentages of women than would be expected were classified as high risk and had their membranes artificially ruptured. A more frequent summoning of paediatricians than is usual was also observed.

Data from the audit also provided further evidence of the lack of continuity of carer during the antenatal period for women in the study group, confirming that the lack of continuity of care for women in the study group was real and not the consequence of difference in reporting by women in the study and control groups.

Evaluation by means of a randomized trial, however scientifically desirable, can be difficult for practical, economic and political reasons. For example, the use of a randomized trial to evaluate a new midwifery led unit at Bournemouth was not thought feasible. Randomizing all the women eligible for booking at the new unit into two groups, one of which would continue to be booked there for delivery and another of which would be delivered at an adjacent consultant unit, would have reduced deliveries at the new unit to the point where it was not viable (Campbell and Macfarlane, 1995). In addition, the unit was opened after a fierce battle (Evans, 1996). It was thought that many local women, who had campaigned so hard to get the unit opened, would refuse to participate in a trial which meant that they had only a fifty per cent chance of being booked for delivery there. In this case a quasi experimental approach was adopted in the evaluation.

Before and after study

As its title suggests, this approach involves taking a variety of measurements prior to a service change and then repeating the same measurements after the service change has had time to settle down. Differences between the measurements at the two points in time are then taken to be the result of the change in service. It is based on an experimental design with the 'before' measurement representing the control group and the 'after' measurement the intervention or experimental group.

This design was used by Sara Twaddle and colleagues (Twaddle et al., 1993) to evaluate a change from a traditional system of postnatal home visiting by community midwives involving a visit on every day until the tenth day, to a pattern of visits based on individual women's needs.

Before there were any discussions with community midwives about individualizing care, baseline data about the postnatal service were collected by reviewing case notes and from questionnaires to midwives and women. An action plan consisting of aims and objectives for individualizing care was then drawn up in discussion with home based midwives. Three months after the new system of care had been introduced more data were collected. Details of the different types of data collected and the sources can be found in Box 4.5.

Box 4.5: Data collected before and after and its source	
Demographic and clinical characteristics of women	Hospital records
Postnatal problems recorded by midwives	Kardex
Postnatal problems reported by women	Self completed questionnaire
Postnatal hospital admission (babies and mothers)	Hospital records
Advice calls received	Log kept by midwives at hospital
Details of postnatal care including day of discharge from hospital, number of postnatal visits and number of midwives visiting	Home based midwife records and an additional midwifery record completed after the final visit
Views of women	Self completed questionnaire
Views of midwives	Self completed questionnaire – before Discussions groups – after
Cost of community midwifery service	Administrative records
(Source: Twaddle et al., 1993)	

One of the potential problems with this method is that the women at the two stages may differ in ways which could have produced differences in outcome. Checks by the researchers, however, indicated that there were no differences between the women in age, parity, mode of delivery or type of postnatal problems.

The results suggested the new pattern of care was efficacious. Individualizing care led to a reduction in the number of postnatal visits from 6.5 to 5.7 and continuity of carer was increased with the average number of different midwives seen dropping from 3.7 to 2.5. Women appeared to be satisfied with both the traditional and individualized pattern of care, but a smaller proportion of those who received individualized care thought that daily visits were necessary.

It was calculated that the normal load of visits might be reduced by ten per cent. The change to individualized care was accompanied by a very small increase in the number of in-patient days. In the economic evaluation three possible scenarios were suggested:

1. Number of postnatal visits decreases but visits take longer so only costs saving on travelling expenses.
2. Fewer postnatal visits result in time being freed up for other activities such as more antenatal clinics and health promotion activities. Cost savings on travelling expenses but costs may be incurred as a result of other activities.
3. Fewer visits but time free not used for other activities. Costs saving on travelling expenses in short term and in longer term saving on midwives' salaries if number of midwife hours reduced.

The researchers argued that the first two scenarios would result in cost effectiveness because women would receive higher quality care for a slightly reduced cost. They suggested that the emphasis on the extended role of the midwife made the third scenario the least likely.

Qualitative evaluation

All of the approaches considered to date in this chapter have involved quantitative methods but qualitative methods can also be employed to particularly good effect in larger scale evaluations. They can be used in tandem with quantitative methods or on their own. Jo Green and colleagues used an ethnographic approach, involving observations and interviews, in a study to evaluate the effect of removing the registrar grade from the medical staffing structure of hospital obstetric units (Green, Kitzinger and Coupland, 1994).

The aim of the first stage of this study was fairly loosely defined as being to 'examine midwives' and doctors' roles and relations in three hospitals which had no obstetric registrars and three with a traditional staffing structure'. This stage was followed up by a large prospective survey of women who gave birth in all of these units, in order to explore their expectations and experiences of childbirth.

The field work undertaken is itemized in Box 4.6. Major themes were identified from all the notes from observations and interviews when the researchers re-read them all after the field work was complete. Some of these themes arose from questions posed by the researchers in the interviews but others had not been anticipated prior to the data collection. All sections of the interviews and observation notes were then categorized according to the themes identified. From these the researchers were able to identify 'predominant attitudes and arrive at some conclusions about majority views'. In order to test the generalizability of their initial findings, the researchers also collected supplementary data on roles and responsibilities from another nine units, one of which did not have registrars (two tier units).

Box 4.6: Field work (stage 1)

Interviews: 18 consultants
                         30 SHOs and registrars
                         85 midwives

Informal discussions took place with a further 79 midwives

Observations
Three researchers spent over 400 hours observing in the labour ward. Half of this time was at night or weekends.

(Source: Green et al., 1986)

In order to maintain the anonymity of the units involved, each unit was given a fictitious name in reports of the findings. In these reports typical attitudes were often illustrated with a verbatim quote but divergent views were also reported.

The researchers had expected to find midwives having an extended role where registrars were absent. They did find midwives more likely to undertake suturing and the topping up of epidurals in units without registrars, but when all the hospitals were considered, they could not find a clear association between the staffing structure and the range of tasks performed by midwives. Not surprisingly, the work did show that consultants were much more involved in the activities of the labour ward when registrars were not part of the staff complement and that midwives were more likely to make decisions. The relationships between doctors and midwives varied according to the medical staffing structure. In two tier units the relationship between the consultants and midwives tended to be closer and more respectful but Senior House Officers were more dissatisfied because they felt the increase in the status of midwives had been to their detriment.

In each of the units studied, a clear set of values and attitudes held by the majority of the permanent staff working there emerged. The researchers characterized the ethos in four of the units as follows:

- Willowford (two tier): 'Active birth – midwives rule OK'
- Wychester (two tier): 'Women's right to choose'
- Exington (three tier): 'The consultants rule the roost'
- Zedbury (three tier): 'Who'd have been responsible if he'd dropped it?'

Only a qualitative approach could have revealed the individual ethos of each unit. This proved to be very important because the results of the surveys in the second phase of the study showed that women were more satisfied with the care they received if they had delivered in units which had a more women centred ethos. These units also happened to be the two tier units. The researchers concluded that while the unit ethos could operate independently from the staffing structure, the two tier structure was more likely to lead to a more empathetic approach to childbearing.

As indicated at the beginning of this chapter, most of the more comprehensive evaluations described here required considerable resourcing and planning. It is important that some evaluations are tackled in this way, particularly when major new ways of organizing care are being implemented. Many useful evaluations can, nevertheless, be undertaken on a smaller scale focusing on one or two rather than a whole panoply of maternity service goals. Ways of doing so are discussed in the next five chapters.

References

Brocklehurst, P., Macfarlane, A., Duley, L., Garcia, G., Elbourne, D. (1995). 'Conclusions are not supported by results'. (Letter). *BMJ*, Vol. 310, p. 806.

Campbell, R., Macfarlane, A. (1995). *Evaluation of the Midwife-led Maternity Unit at the Royal Bournemouth Hospital.* Preliminary report. Report to the Dorset Health Commission. Oxford: National Perinatal Epidemiology Unit.

Department of Health (1995). *Improving the Health of Mothers and Children: NHS Priorities for Research and Development.* London: Department of Health.

Evans, J. (1996). 'Supporting a local midwife led service – Bournemouth Maternity Unit'. Paper presented at a Changing Childbirth Regional Conference, Weston Super Mare.

Farquhar, M., Camilleri-Ferrante, C., Todd, C. (1996). 'An evaluation of midwifery teams in West Essex'. University of Cambridge: Public health Resources Unit & Health Services Research Group, Institute of Public Health.

Green, J., Kitzinger, J., Coupland, V. (1986). *The Division of Labour: Implications of Medical Staffing Structures for Midwives and Doctors on the Labour Ward.* Cambridge: Childcare and Development Group.

Green, J., Kitzinger, J., Coupland, V. (1994). 'Midwives' responsibilities, medical staffing structures and women's choice in childbirth'. In: Robinson, S., Thomson, A.M. (Eds). *Midwives, Research and Childbirth.* London: Chapman Hall.

Hundley, V. Personal communication.

Hundley, V., Cruickshank, F., Lang, G. et al. (1994). 'Midwife managed delivery unit: a randomised controlled comparison with consultant led care'. *BMJ*, Vol. 309, pp. 1400–1404.

Hundley, V.A., Cruickshank, F.M., Milne J.M. et al. (1995a). 'Satisfaction and continuity of care: staff views of care in a midwife-managed delivery unit'. *Midwifery*, Vol. 11, pp. 163–173.

Hundley, V.A., Donaldson, C., Lang, G.D. et al. (1995b). 'Costs of intrapartum care in a midwife-managed delivery unit and a consultant-led labour ward'. *Midwifery*, Vol. 11, pp. 103–109.

Rowley, M.J., Brinamead, M., Hensley, M.J., Wlodarczyk, W. (1995). 'Continuity of care by a midwife team versus routine care during pregnancy and birth: a randomized trial'. *Medical Journal of Australia*, Vol. 163, pp. 289–293.

Newell, D.J. (1992). 'Intention to treat analysis: implications for quantitative and qualitative research'. *International Journal of Epidemiology*, Vol. 21, pp. 837–841.

Smith, L. (1995). Analysis is invalid'. (Letter). *BMJ*, Vol. 310, pp. 805–806.

Twaddle, S., Liao, X.H., Fyvie, H. (1993). 'An evaluation of postnatal care individualised to the needs of the women'. *Midwifery*, Vol. 9, No. 3, pp. 154–160.

CHAPTER FIVE

Finding Out What Women And Their Families Think Of Maternity Services

Jo Garcia

'The changes are brilliant. This time round I felt like a person not a piece of meat.' (A mother of four, living in Humberside)

'I thoroughly enjoyed coming home with the baby I loved, but I was terrified that I should do something wrong and not have anybody to get advice from. My husband was loving and helpful around the house but he knew nothing about babies. We both waited anxiously for the midwife's visit which the interpreter at the hospital had explained would happen in the next few days. She was lovely and included my husband in all that was going on.' (A young woman of Kurdish origin, living in London)

The views of women and families are crucial to the evaluation of care. Many of the recent studies that have looked at new forms of maternity organization have included the views of women using the services (see examples listed in Further Reading at the end of this chapter and the detailed descriptions in Chapter 4). This chapter is about systematic ways of finding out about the experiences and opinions of those who use the service. A range of methods can be used including interviews, self-completion questionnaires, group discussions and observation of care. This chapter leaves out some of the important but 'unsystematic' ways that a maternity service responds to those who use it, like collecting suggestions about care and dealing with complaints because these are not usually used as part of evaluations.

The chapter will look first at the different reasons for doing studies of this kind. Next it will cover the main methodological approaches and the types of results that you get from them. Then there will be a section on ways of getting the views of *all* those who use the service, to try to avoid bias and reach people who may not normally take part in studies.

The different reasons for doing these studies

There are several different reasons for seeking information of this kind, and though they overlap, it is worth considering them in turn.

Probably the most common reason is to help in the audit of care by seeking information that only women who receive it can give, or that is simpler or more reliable to collect from women. For example, studies have asked whether a woman knew the people caring for her at particular times, whether she was given information about services or about her health, whether she tried to contact her midwife by phone, whether appointments were convenient, whether she brought her children to the clinic, or what sort of classes she went to. Some examples of this type of question are shown in Box 5.1. They all come from self-completion questionnaires.

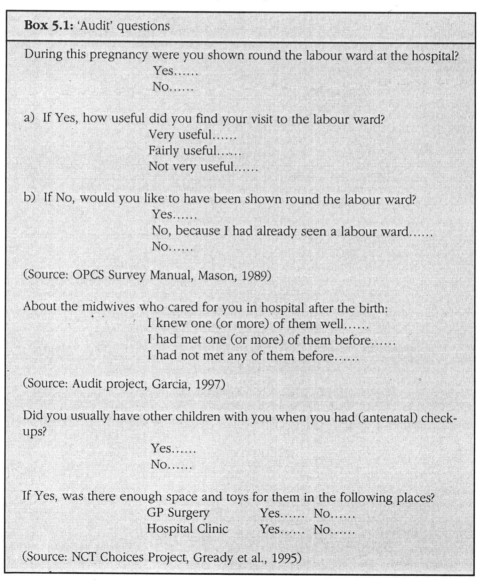

Box 5.1: 'Audit' questions

During this pregnancy were you shown round the labour ward at the hospital?
        Yes......
        No......

a) If Yes, how useful did you find your visit to the labour ward?
        Very useful......
        Fairly useful......
        Not very useful......

b) If No, would you like to have been shown round the labour ward?
        Yes......
        No, because I had already seen a labour ward......
        No......

(Source: OPCS Survey Manual, Mason, 1989)

About the midwives who cared for you in hospital after the birth:
        I knew one (or more) of them well......
        I had met one (or more) of them before......
        I had not met any of them before......

(Source: Audit project, Garcia, 1997)

Did you usually have other children with you when you had (antenatal) check-ups?
        Yes......
        No......

If Yes, was there enough space and toys for them in the following places?
        GP Surgery   Yes...... No......
        Hospital Clinic   Yes...... No......

(Source: NCT Choices Project, Gready et al., 1995)

Very closely tied in to these sort of 'audit' questions are another type of question about how a woman felt about the care, and whether it met her needs. The dividing line isn't always clear. The sort of topics covered include whether the woman got the information she wanted, whether her views were taken into account, or whether she was treated kindly. She can be asked about conflicting advice, about fears and anxieties and about how helpful the care was. Some questions ask about her satisfaction with care. Examples of this type of question are given in Box 5.2. There is also the possibility of asking about 'housekeeping' issues that are important, particularly in postnatal care in hospital – questions about food, cleanliness, telephones, visiting times and so on. All these questions could be called *evaluative* because they ask someone to assess and comment on the care.

Box 5.2: Evaluative questions

How would you describe the way the staff looked after you during your labour and the birth?

> Kind and understanding all the time......
> Kind and understanding most of the time......
> Kind and understanding sometimes......
> Never kind and understanding......

(Source: NCT Choices Project, Gready et al., 1995)

During labour and delivery, did you feel that the midwives were too busy to spend enough time with you?

> Yes, often too busy......
> Yes, sometimes too busy......
> No, not really......

(Source: OPCS Survey Manual, Mason, 1989)

From a questionnaire for women at around 34 weeks of pregnancy:

a) During your pregnancy, do you feel that overall you have been given:
> Too much information......
> The right amount of information......
> Too little information......
> Too much about some things, too little about others......

b) Is there anything in particular that you wish you had known more about?

> Yes......   No......   Don't know......

> if Yes, what?......

From a questionnaire sent when the baby was a few weeks old:

Have any of the tests that your baby has had caused you any anxiety?
> Yes...... No......
> if Yes, please tell us about it.

(Source: Both questionnaires come from a study by Jo Green and colleagues about screening in maternity care (Statham and Green, 1994)

Audit and evaluative questions are often combined in studies carried out within maternity services. Studies of this kind can be very useful, especially if they are well focused, if they ask about things that are of concern to care givers, and if there is a commitment to act on the results. Here are one or two examples from the very large number of studies (Box 5.3).

Box 5.3: Examples of studies by providers

King's College Hospital – Regular surveys of women who have recently given birth

Six surveys of women's views have now been carried out at King's in south London. The questionnaire has been modified somewhat since the first survey in 1991, for example to take into account issues raised by the Maternity Services Liaison Committee. This approach has been able to demonstrate improvements in care; for example the proportion of women waiting for more than an hour at the hospital antenatal clinic has fallen from over 50 per cent in April 1991 to around 10 per cent in the survey carried out at the end of 1994. In contrast, there have been signs of a fall in the standard of some aspects of hospital postnatal care, with a small but steady reduction in the numbers of women describing the postnatal ward as welcoming, friendly and helpful. Infant feeding support and advice seems to be getting better. For example, the proportion of women who discussed breastfeeding at antenatal visits and classes has increased steadily over the last three surveys. The results of these surveys are written up by the information midwife and presented to the MSLC and to managers and other staff. They are part of the process of auditing and planning care (Dobson, Personal communication).

A qualitative study in one general practice

This study was carried out in a health centre with six GPs serving nearly 16,000 patients. The aim was to review the care that was given to pregnant women and babies in the practice. Interviews were carried out by an independent researcher with 52 women attending antenatal appointments at the health centre. The interviews were based on a list of topics to be covered and did not include structured questions. In addition two focus groups were convened at a day centre for under-fives and parents. The topics addressed in the interviews and focus groups included access and appointments, contact with midwives and GPs, quality of care and suggestions for improvement. The findings led to some changes in the way that care was provided. For example, antenatal appointments were arranged so that a GP would be available to join the midwife if necessary. Because a few women reported that they were uncomfortable with a home visit by the midwife, the care has been changed so that women are offered this possibility rather than having it routinely (Mellor and Chambers, 1995)

If we step back from the detailed aspects of care we come up with another reason for doing studies of the views of those using the service. Purchasers have the task of trying to find out what sort of services would be desired by the women for whom they are responsible. A number of studies have tried to go beyond women's reactions to their care in order to ascertain what women prefer, or how important different aspects of care are for women. For example, is it more important to women to have care that is convenient, or kind, or from a woman professional? How important is it to get to know the care givers? How much interest do women have in the possibility of a home birth or care in a GP unit? Purchasers also have responsibility for *all women* in an area and so they may need to ask questions about equity and accessibility. Are services conveniently located and accessible to women? Do women know about the options available to them? Are there special needs that some categories of women have, and are these being met? There are some examples of studies of this kind in Box 5.4. It is worth noting that studies about what sort of service women want can be difficult to do mainly because the answers are very much affected by the ways that the questions are phrased.

Box 5.4: Examples of studies by purchasers

Women's experiences of Maternity Services in East London
This study was carried out by the purchasers of maternity services provided by three large inner city hospitals. It used a postal questionnaire to mothers who were resident within the area and who had given birth within a three week period. Women who did not speak English were interviewed by bilingual interviewers. The response rate was 67 per cent (356/533). The study showed important differences in many aspects of the care provided by the three hospitals. For example, the number of women who had more than ten antenatal visits varied from 29 per cent to 56 per cent. The study showed that women who did not have English as their main language were nearly twice as likely to report that they did not have continuity of midwifery carer. The results were used in discussions about the service specifications for the next year and contributed to the agenda of the Maternity Services Liaison Committee (Hemingway et al., 1994).

Women from minority ethnic groups in Leeds
Leeds Family Health Services Authority carried out a study of the views of women from minority ethnic groups about maternity care. It used interviews, self-completion questionnaires and focused discussion groups. The study found that around 40 per cent of women had difficulty in communicating with care givers because of language and many recommended that bilingual workers be employed. Women wanted improved access to female doctors. The study also found that there were aspects of maternity care that some women did not know about or understand. Over 70 per cent of women wanted to know more about hospital tests and procedures (Leeds Family Health, 1992).

There are two other types of studies that are more research oriented and which we will only cover briefly here. Some studies have been carried out where women are the informants about aspects of clinical care and practice. Information from women generally compares well with that from clinical records (e.g. Martin, 1987). These studies are usually national or regional surveys using postal questionnaires, and are either epidemiological (concerned with risks and health outcomes) or concerned with policy making. Some examples are described briefly in Box 5.5. A national survey of a random sample of mothers in England and Wales was carried out by the Audit Commission in 1996 and used in their report on maternity services (Audit Commission, 1997).

Box 5.5: National or regional surveys

The dignity of labour?

This classic study was carried out in 1975 by Ann Cartwright. Nearly 2500 recently delivered women in England and Wales were interviewed about their experience of labour and birth. The study covered a wide range of topics but focused particularly on induction of labour and on the experience of women who had had a stillbirth. The many useful results of this study include evidence of wide variation in some aspects of care. For example, when the 37 hospitals with more than 20 deliveries in the sample were compared, it was found that the proportion of women whose husbands were present at some point during labour and delivery varied from 20% to 95%. The study was important in the debate about induction and other interventions and came at a crucial time for change in maternity care. The findings also emphasized women's needs for information about all aspects of their maternity care (Cartwright, 1979).

Survey of recent mothers in Victoria, Australia

This was a postal questionnaire study of all women giving birth in Victoria in one week in 1989, as part of a review of birthing services commissioned by the state's health department. The questionnaires were sent out when the babies were 8–9 months old and were returned by 790 women. A follow-up study of women who were depressed (and random controls) was carried out using home interviews. The study explored many familiar issues about the quality of personal care and women's needs for good information and communication with care givers, and put the findings into the context of the patterns of care available locally. Of particular interest is the authors' work on postnatal depression. They found that in their study population one woman in seven was depressed according to the definition they used, and so they returned to as many of them as possible to find out more about it. Very few studies have asked women about their experience of depression. Women in this study described what it was like to be depressed, what help they had looked for and what help they had received from partners, health care workers and lay groups (Brown et al., 1994).

Pain relief in labour – a UK study

This study was carried out by researchers for the National Birthday Trust Fund and covered all births in the UK in one week in 1990. The aim was to provide a picture of facilities and to get the views of women, partners and staff about different approaches to pain relief in labour. Questionnaires to women just after the birth and at six weeks after delivery provided part of the data. The study was large and complex and involved over 10,000 women. It collected unique data about women's assessments of the various methods of pain relief. The data collected at six weeks after the birth provide useful information about women's health and their views of the care they received (Chamberlain, Wraight and Steer, 1993).

The second type of research-oriented approach is intended to increase understanding of childbearing in society, and is not set up (initially, at least) to provide information that is of day-to-day use to the health service. Again, these studies do not divide themselves neatly from some of the others above and many of them *are* of great value to those concerned with maternity care. The researchers, who usually have a background in psychology or sociology, are seeking to understand childbearing and parenthood, sometimes in the context of health care, but often in a wider setting. The small number of studies of the views of fathers are nearly all of this type. The studies under this heading are very diverse and a few are shown in Box 5.6 to illustrate the range.

Box 5.6: The social context of maternity care

Mothers under twenty
Teenage motherhood is often seen as a problem, but how is it viewed by young mothers themselves? This study interviewed women aged between 16 and 19 who had babies in 1985–6 and explored their views about themselves and their ideas about parenthood. Women in this study were aware that young mothers were seen in a negative light, but often defined themselves in a way that excluded these problems. The cut off at 20 was seen as rather arbitrary by many of them and some mentioned that they did not feel like particularly young mothers because many of their friends had had babies even younger. The study explored the arguments that these women drew on to explain and justify their current role and in the process helps to illuminate society's ideas about mothers and motherhood (Phoenix, 1991).

Becoming a mother
This is a key study for those interested in understanding maternity care and women's roles in society. It was carried out by Ann Oakley in 1975–6 and involved interviews with 66 women expecting their first babies and booked at one London hospital. Each women was interviewed four times, twice before the birth and twice after, and the interviews were tape recorded. These data were used in preparing two books, one focusing on the academic debates and issues and the other giving most of its space to women's accounts of their experiences. The study led Ann Oakley to further work in this field and also prompted a great deal of debate and interest (Oakley, 1979, 1980).

Fathers and maternity care
This small-scale study aimed to look at the involvement of fathers antenatally, in labour and after the birth. It is based on interviews with 18 couples and observation of care in several maternity hospitals. It provided interesting insights into the ways that fathers see themselves, and are seen by women and midwives. Fathers who expressed a reluctance to be present at the birth were seen as deviant in this study, though the reasons given for wanting them to be there varied considerably between women. Their participation in baby care on the postnatal ward was minimal in some places, but substantial in others perhaps reflecting the evolution of family centred policies about babies and children in hospital (Barbour, 1990).

The range of methods

There is a wide range of methods used to obtain the views of women about care that they have experienced or that they would like. Most studies use self-completion questionnaires, but interviews, group discussions and observation have also been used. Although there is discussion and debate about the relative merits of the different approaches, or different styles of questionnaire, there is not much published work that addresses these methodological issues in relation to maternity care.

In Table 5.1 there are examples of studies in the maternity field that use the different methods, and some reference books that may be useful. Quite a few studies use more than one method, for example, a small scale interview study initially to get an idea of the range of issues that people are concerned about, followed by a postal questionnaire to a larger number in order get a more representative picture. The number of people that you include in a study affects the sort of conclusions that you can draw. If you want to make statistical comparisons of the breastfeeding rate in two parts of your area, for example, you need to calculate an appropriate sample size (for a discussion on sample sizes for surveys see Crombie and Davies, 1996, Chapter 6). In order to generalize from your sample to the wider population it is important to think about possible sources of bias. For example, if you want to know whether women find the time of community based antenatal classes convenient you need to ask all possible attenders and not just those who already come.

Which method to use?

The choice of method depends on:

* what the study is trying to do;
* what is already known about the topic;
* practicalities;
* the resources available.

Since there is only limited guidance about which methods work well in which circumstances, decisions are often based on experience and common sense. Table 5.1 sets out some of the strengths and weaknesses of the various approaches.

How should one go about deciding which method is appropriate? Here are two examples. You are concerned about an aspect of care that affects only a very few women coming through your service – care for women having a late termination for suspected fetal abnormality. The method most likely to be useful would probably be based on interviews with families who have undergone a late termination. The interviews would be fairly open and would cover issues specific to the local service. In addition to getting detailed information about what the care was like, they could allow parents to raise continuing worries and uncertainties and be guided to seek information from the appropriate part of the service. It would not be an easy job to design, carry out and analyse these interviews but advice and help should be available from local academic departments of social sciences.

METHOD	PROS AND CONS	EXAMPLES FROM MATERNITY CARE	USEFUL GENERAL REFERENCES
interviews	**pro:** • flexible • good for difficult or complex topics • good for smaller samples • can be more or less structured **con:** • slower or more expensive	Cartwright, 1979 Oakley, 1979, 1980, 1992 Brown et al., 1994	Mays and Pope, 1996 Morse and Field, 1996
self-administered questionnaire	**pro:** • cheaper • easier to analyse • can be anonymous • helps generalizability **con:** • poorer/no response from some • sections of population • 'shallow' • researcher's agenda	Cartwright, 1986 Oakley, 1992 Green et al., 1990 McHaffie, 1996 Gready et al., 1995 Brown et al., 1994 There are a great many other studies using this method	Cartwright, 1983 Crombie and Davies, 1996 (Chap 6)
focus groups	**pro:** • allows new themes to be raised • can be cheaper than interviews **con:** • practical difficulties – hard to get participants • some opinions may not be voiced • usually small scale	Mellor and Chambers, 1995 Gready et al., 1995 N. Derbyshire Health Authority, 1991 There are not many published examples of focus group studies in maternity care	Kreuger, 1988 Kitzinger, 1995 Morgan, 1993
observation	**pro:** • a chance to see 'real' behaviour • can show gaps between views and actions **con:** • demanding for researcher • can alter behaviour • limited generalizability	Kirkham, 1983, 1989 Garcia & Garforth, 1990 Hunt & Symonds, 1995 Barbour, 1990 Bowler, 1993 a, b. Again, there are only a small number of observation studies in maternity care	Mays and Pope, 1996 Fielding, 1993

Table 5.1: Some methods for getting people's views

A different method might be appropriate to help solve the next problem. Midwives are concerned about the care of mothers living in an area with a lot of short term accommodation. They feel that women are missing antenatal visits and are not easy to reach after the birth because so many move. You could set up some meetings with women in the area. These meetings would aim to find out what the problems were from the point of view of the women, what needs they express and what they think of the solutions that you have in mind. Meetings of this kind may be particularly useful when you are looking for ideas about change. It is not always easy to set them up and you need guidance from someone with experience of organizing and running the meetings and using the information collected.

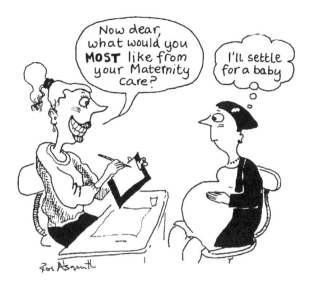

Reaching women

An issue for any type of method, but particularly surveys, is that those who may have a great deal to tell us about care are least likely to respond to questionnaires or take part in discussions. In general, women who are poorer, younger and more mobile are less likely to participate in research studies (e.g. Mason 1989; Cartwright 1986; Brown et al.,1994). In addition, many studies do not enable non-English speaking women to take part. There are ways of trying to remedy these deficiencies. Some studies have used small groups to learn about the needs of particular categories of women. For example in the Choices project carried out in Essex (Gready et al., 1995), a postal survey was complemented by focus groups with women who had special experiences or needs – for example, bereaved women and young women. Face-to-face recruitment may improve the response rates for some studies. In a study of postnatal care, women who were approached in person by the research midwife were more likely to send back questionnaires than women who were written to (Marchant, personal communication). There are studies about aspects of questionnaire design and survey methods which can help to improve response rates. Experience with questionnaire design and analysis can help to make the questions readable, clear and easy to analyse. Some issues that arise for non English-speaking women are covered in the next section.

Assessing the needs and experiences of women using the maternity services who do not speak or write English

If you want to know what women think of the maternity services in your area you may find that there are women whose views you are interested in but who do not take part in surveys or come to open meetings. For some women this is because English is not their first language, so they cannot use the questionnaire or do not feel confident about taking part. They may not be literate in their own language. Many non-English speaking women in this country come from Asia or Africa, but there are also refugees from Europe and South America living in some areas.

Recent studies (e.g. Rudat et al., 1993) estimate that nationally about 40 per cent of women between 16–35 of Bangladeshi origin do not speak English. For women from Pakistan the same figure is 29 per cent and 13 per cent for women of Indian origin. In East London the proportions of women who speak little or no English in these age groups are high – 64 per cent for women of Bangladeshi origin, 56 per cent of Turkish and Kurdish women and 37 per cent of women of Chinese background. This shows that there is likely to be a substantial need for interpreting services, though it may be very localized, and may well shift over time. There are many advocacy, interpreting or liaison schemes and these are based in maternity units and in the community. Large, well established minority ethnic groups may be easier to cater for than rapidly changing, diverse communities with small numbers of women from many different backgrounds.

Good quality maternity care is almost impossible if no help is provided for those women who do not speak English. Those who are involved in the provision or planning of care need to know about needs and about women's views of care. The changes that are taking place in the organization of maternity services need to be assessed from the viewpoint of *all* women, including those who do not use English. In addition any special services should be evaluated and adapted to changing needs and to the general changes in service organization. For example, if there is a shift to community-based care then the way that help is provided for women who need interpreters or advocates may need to be reassessed.

Although there has not been a great deal of work to compare what you get from the various approaches to assessing the views of health service users, there is a consensus about the most practical approaches for women from non-English speaking backgrounds. In general self-administered postal questionnaires in English do not work well. Translated questionnaires have been used in a few projects, and may be successful in some communities. The view of researchers is, however, that the poor response that is usually obtained with this approach makes it inappropriate. In one Australian study of maternity services, the offer of a questionnaire translated into Vietnamese or Arabic was taken up by only one person (Brown et al., 1994). Other methods are available. In the field of maternity care, interesting studies have been done using interpreted interviews, bilingual interviewers, focused group discussions and direct observation of care. Some examples are given in Box 5.7.

The choice of method for getting the views of women who do not speak English depends on the question being addressed, and on practical considerations like cost. If, for example, the aim is to set up and assess a local scheme to provide access to female doctors at out-patient visits then focus groups would be a good first step. These would give an idea of the demand and look at the practical aspects of provision. Assessment of the new scheme might use a simple questionnaire administered by bilingual interviewers. If, on the other hand, there was a need for data to inform the national policy agenda about the maternity provision for Black and Asian women, then a larger (more costly) study would be needed. In one such study, own-language interviews were carried out with a national sample of 300 Black and Asian women (Rudat et al., 1993). The questionnaire was almost identical to that used for interviews with a larger national random sample of women, so that comparisons could then be made between the experiences and views of the minority ethnic group sample and of the mainly white, national random sample.

Box 5.7: Studies of maternity care for women in minority ethnic groups

A small scale study using observation and interviews in a maternity hospital
The data are drawn from a small-scale ethnographic study which investigated Asian women's maternity experience by using observation on the labour ward, in the antenatal clinic and in the community as well as in formal interviews. The midwives' views about Asian women were found to contain four main themes: the difficulty of communicating with the women; the women's lack of compliance with care and abuse of the service; their tendency to 'make a fuss about nothing'; and their lack of 'normal maternal instinct'. Stereotyping reflected and reinforced the view that Asian women are 'all the same' but 'not like us'. Midwives used stereotypes to help them to make judgements about the kind of care different women wanted, needed and deserved. It is therefore argued that stereotyping is a factor in the creation of the inequality in health experiences of black and minority ethnic patients. The section on communication difficulties is particularly illuminating, showing how misunderstandings arise and how difficult it is for women with little English to make a personal relationship with the midwives and therefore challenge the assumptions made about them (Bowler, 1993a, b).

Home interviews carried out by a bilingual researcher
In this study 32 Asian women living in East London were interviewed by an Asian woman psychologist to assess their views and experiences of childbirth and postnatal care. The women were recruited from GP surgeries and through subsequent contacts and were interviewed in English, Hindi, Punjabi or Urdu. The interviews were semi-structured. Women varied in terms of their parity, time since delivery, religion and social class. Some had been born and educated in the UK, the others had come as adults and lived here for varying lengths of time. A significant part of their accounts concerned their experiences in the postnatal wards. Their concerns in many ways reflected those previously reported by non-Asian women but a number of additional issues were raised. These included the importance of rest and recovery and the feeling that staff expected too much of mothers in the early postnatal days. They were less preoccupied with the issue of mother-infant bonding than with the impact of the birth on the whole family. Many of the English speaking women expressed concern about the quality of care given to non-English speakers, though these women themselves reported few difficulties or tensions with staff (Woollett and Dosanjh-Matwala, 1990).

There are practical and methodological difficulties in work in this area. The choice of methods is not straightforward, the research is often quite expensive and researchers do not always succeed in getting the co-operation of the communities concerned. Funding bodies may be less willing to consider studies that use qualitative methods, because they are seen as 'soft'. For these reasons, research should not be embarked upon too hastily. Is research needed? Can the results of relevant work elsewhere be applied here? It is important to search out experienced researchers and useful (often unpublished) projects by making contact with some of the places listed in Box 5.8.

If, however, it is clear that research is needed, then appropriate research methods are not a luxury. They are crucial to enabling the views of some sectors of the population to be heard.

Box 5.8: Resources for studies of maternity care for minority ethnic groups

---

Organizations:
Share Project, based at the King's Fund, 11–13 Cavendish Square. London W1M 0AN. Newsletter, subject based bibliographies and contacts (Tel: 0171 307 2400)

Department of Health: Department's Advisor on Ethnic Minority Health, Ms Veena Bahl, Department of Health, Wellington House, 133–155 Waterloo Rd, London SE1 8UG (Tel: 0171 972 4671)

Changing Childbirth Team, Health Care and Public Health Directorate, NHS Executive Anglia and Oxford, 6–12 Capital Drive, Linford Wood, Milton Keynes, MK14 6QP (Tel: 01908 844400)

Maternity Alliance, 45 Beech St, 5th Floor, London EC2P 2LX (Tel: 0171 588 8583)

Useful publications:
McIver, S. (1994). *Obtaining the Views of Black Users of the Health Services.* London, Kings Fund (Copies from BEBC, for information freephone 0800–262260)

Health Education Authority (1994). *Health Related Resources for Black and Minority Ethnic Groups* and (1995) *Health and Lifestyle Survey: Black and Minority Ethnic Groups in England.* HEA (Tel: 0171 383 3833)

Commission for Racial Equality (1994). *Race Relations Code of Practice in Maternity Services.* London: Commission for Racial Equality (Tel: 0171 828 7022)

Dodds, R., Goodman, M., Tyler, S. (1996). *Listen with Mother: Consulting Users of the Maternity Services.* Hale, Cheshire: Books for Midwives Press.

People from minority ethnic backgrounds rightly point out that research is an unjustified imposition on those who take part if there is no real commitment to take the results into account. This, though, is true for all members of the public who take the time to write about their care, fill in a questionnaire or come to a meeting. Research of this kind takes up people's time and uses public resources. There is an ethical obligation, therefore, only to do research that is needed and where there is a good chance that the results will be used, and to do the work as well as possible. Research approaches are about getting a systematic, up to date and unbiased view of women's needs and experiences. Without the representation of service users on bodies that have power to make changes, research findings may linger on the shelf, or may be applied in a very limited way (NHS Executive, 1996). Consultation with community organizations and representatives will complement research and be crucial to implementing change.

Interpreting the results

Finally there are some issues about interpreting the results of studies of service users.

Are the results representative? This has been referred to already. If some people do not respond to a survey how do we judge whether to make changes in a service on the basis of the views that we do have? There are no rules here, but common sense can take us quite a long way. If the response rate is very low, then it may be that those who *did* respond had very good or bad experiences. We should be cautious about making changes on the basis of the results. If the data show that women from some areas are under-represented then it would be wise to find other sources of information before altering the times of a class, or the siting of a clinic in that area.

Making comparisons is tempting but needs caution. It can be risky to make judgements about the relative quality of services in two places by comparing the views expressed by those who use them. This is particularly a problem where evaluative questions are used. For example, women in one place may have different expectations from those in another, so questions about how good information or communications were, may be answered differently, even where services were similar. When comparisons are made over time in the same place, this caveat also applies, but it is probably sensible to have confidence that we are seeing real changes, when such changes are found between surveys that are not too far apart. This makes more sense if we imagine using the same questions separated by ten or fifteen years. We would certainly be cautious about ascribing any changes that we saw to changes only in the service.

The same caution applies to making comparisons within the data from a survey. If, for example, women within a service have had antenatal care from two types of care giver we may want to compare their experience of audit type items such as waiting times and convenience of appointments, but because they are likely to have been self-selected to some extent, we should be careful about comparing satisfaction on other more evaluative aspects of the questionnaire. The other way to put this is to say that we can only rarely draw cause and effect conclusions from studies of women's views. If we want to be more confident that a change in the service has led to a particular outcome, then randomized controlled trials are needed (see Chapters 3 and 4). These issues of interpretation were discussed at a conference organized by several maternity groups. This led to a useful book called *Listen with Mother* (Dodds et al., 1996).

Getting good advice

In spite of the great interest in women's views of care, and the changes that have been taking place in the services, there has not been an attempt to produce a basic core questionnaire for maternity since the OPCS Survey Manual (Mason, 1989). Two short versions of the OPCS questionnaire have been produced and tested (Hemingway et al., 1994; Lamping and Rowe, 1996). The College of Health is producing a resource pack which will contain basic sets of questions and guidance on ways of getting women's views (for further information contact the College of Health on 0181 983 1225). The Changing Childbirth Team may also be able to help by putting you in touch with other people doing evaluations (see Box 5.8 for the address).

References

Audit Commission (1997). *First Class Delivery. Improving Maternity Services in England and Wales*. London: Audit Commission.

Barbour, R. (1990). 'Fathers: the emergence of a new consumer group'. In: Garcia, J., Kilpatrick, R., Richards, M. (Eds.). *The Politics of Maternity Care*. Oxford: Oxford University Press.

Bowler, I. (1993a). '"They're not the same as us": midwives' stereotypes of South Asian descent maternity patients'. *Sociology of Health & Illness,* Vol. 15, No. 2, pp. 157–178.

Bowler, I. (1993b). 'Stereotypes of women of Asian descent in midwifery: some evidence'. *Midwifery,* Vol. 9, No. 1, pp. 7–16.

Brown, S., Lumley, J., Small, R., Astbury, J. (1994). *Missing Voices; The Experience of Motherhood*. Oxford: Oxford University Press.

Cartwright, A. (1979). *The Dignity of Labour?* London: Tavistock.

Cartwright, A. (1983). *Health Surveys in Practice and Potential: A Critical Review of their Scope and Methods*. London: King Edward's Hospital Fund for London.

Cartwright, A. (1986). 'Who responds to postal questionnaires?'. *Journal of Epidemiology and Community Health,* Vol. 40, pp. 267–73.

Chamberlain, G., Wraight, A., Steer, P. (1993). *Pain and its Relief in Childbirth*. Edinburgh: Churchill Livingstone.

Commission for Racial Equality (1994). *Race Relations Code of Practice in Maternity Services*. London: Commission for Racial Equality.

Crombie and Davies (1996*). Research in Health Care: Design, Conduct and Interpretation of Health Services Research*. Chichester: John Wiley.

Dobson, P. Personal communication.

Dodds, R., Goodman, M., Tyler, S. (1996). *Listen with Mother: Consulting Users of Maternity Services*. Hale, Cheshire: Books for Midwives Press.

Fielding, N. (1993). *Researching Social Life*. London: Sage.

Garcia, J., Garforth, S. (1990). 'Parents and new-born babies in the labour ward'. In: Garcia, J., Richards, M., Kilpatrick, R. (Eds). *The Politics of Maternity Care*. Oxford: Oxford University Press.

Garcia, J. (1997). *Changing Midwifery Care –The Scope for Evaluation: Report of an NHSE-Funded Project*. Oxford: National Perinatal Epidemiology Unit.

Gready, M., Newburn, M., Dodds, R., Gauge, S. (1995). *Birth Choices: Women's Expectations and Experiences*. London: National Childbirth Trust.

Health Education Authority (1994). *Health Related Resources for Black and Minority Ethnic Groups*. London: HEA.

Hemingway, H., Saunders, D., Parsons, L. (1994). *Women's Experiences of Maternity Services in East London: An Evaluation*. London: East London and City Health Authority.

Hunt, S., Symonds, A., (1995). *The Social Meaning of Midwifery*. London: Macmillan.

Kirkham, M. (1983). 'Labouring in the dark – limitations on the giving of information to enable patients to orient themselves to the likely events and timescale of labour'. In: Wilson-Barnett, J. (Ed). *Nursing Research: Ten Studies in Patient Care*. Chichester: John Wiley.

Kirkham, M. (1989). 'Midwives and information-giving in labour'. In: Robinson, S., Thomson, A. (Eds). *Midwives, Research and Childbirth. Vol. I.* London: Chapman and Hall.

Kitzinger, J. (1995). 'Introducing focus groups'. *British Medical Journal,* Vol. 311, pp. 299–302.

Kreuger, R. (1988). *Focus Groups: A Practical Guide for Applied Research*. London: Sage.

Lamping, D., Rowe, P. (1996). *Surveys of Women's Experiences of Maternity Services (Short Form). Users' Manual for Purchasers and Providers*. London: London School of Hygiene and Tropical Medicine.

Leeds Family Health (1992). *Research into the Uptake of Maternity Services as Provided by Primary Health Care Teams to Women from Black and Ethnic Minorities*. Leeds: Leeds FSHA.

McHaffie, H. (1996). 'Supporting families with a very low birthweight baby'. In: Robinson, S., Thomson, A. (Eds). *Midwives, Research and Childbirth. Vol. 4.* London: Chapman and Hall.

McIver, C. (1994). *Obtaining the Views of Black Users of the Health Services.* London: Kings Fund (copies from BEBC; for information freephone 0800-262260).

Martin, C. (1987). 'Monitoring maternity services by postal questionnaire: congruity between mothers' reports and their obstetric records'. *Statistics in Medicine*, Vol. 6, pp. 613–627.

Mason, V. (1989). *Women's Experience of Maternity Care – A Survey Manual.* London: HMSO.

Mays, N., Pope, C. (1996). *Qualitative Research in Health Care.* London: BMJ Publishing Group.

Mellor, J., Chambers, N. (1995). 'Addressing the patient's agenda in the reorganisation of antenatal and infant health care: experience in one general practice'. *British Journal of General Practice*, Vol. 45, pp. 423–425.

Morgan, D. (1993). *Successful Focus Groups: Advancing the State of the Art.* London: Sage.

Morse, J.M., Field, P.A. (1996). *Nursing Research: the Application of Qualitative Approaches.* 2nd Edition. London: Chapman and Hall.

NHS Executive (1996). *Maternity Services Liaison Committees: Guidelines for Working Effectively.* Leeds: NHS Executive.

North Derbyshire Health Authority (1991). *What Kind of Maternity Care do You Want? Results of a Priority Search Survey of 721 Women Living in North Derbyshire.* North Derbyshire Health Authority.

Oakley, A. (1979). *Becoming a Mother.* Oxford: Martin Robertson.

Oakley, A. (1980). *Women Confined: Towards a Sociology of Childbirth.* Oxford: Martin Robertson.

Oakley, A. (1992). *Social Support and Motherhood.* Oxford: Blackwell.

Phoenix, A. (1991). *Young Mothers?* Cambridge: Polity Press.

Rudat, K., Roberts, C., Chowdhury, R. (1993). *Maternity Services: A Comparative Survey of Afro-Caribbean, Asian and White Women Commissioned by the Expert Maternity Group.* MORI Health Research: London.

Statham, H., Green, J. (1994). 'The effects of miscarriage and other "unsuccessful" pregnancies on feelings early in subsequent pregnancies'. *Journal of Reproduction and Infant Psychology*, Vol. 12, pp. 45–54.

Woollett, A., Dosanjh-Matwala, N. (1990). 'Postnatal care: the attitudes and experiences of Asian women in east London'. *Midwifery*, Vol. 6, pp. 178–184.

Further reading

Allen, I., Bourke Dowling, S., Williams, S. (1997). *A Leading Role for Midwives.* London: Policy Studies Institute.

Chapman, M., Roberts, E., Aherne, V., Harrison, A., Morgan, A. (1996). *An Evaluation of Stockport Maternity Services.* Manchester: North West Surveys and Research.

Farquhar, M., Camilleri-Ferrante, C., Todd, C. (1996). *An Evaluation of Midwifery Teams in West Essex.* Cambridge: Public Health Resources Unit & Health Services Research Group, Institute of Public Health, University of Cambridge.

Green, J., Kitzinger, J., Coupland, V. (1994). 'Midwives' responsibilities, medical staffing structures and women's choice in childbirth'. In: Robinson, S., Thomson, A.M. (Eds). *Midwives, Research and Childbirth.* London: Chapman Hall.

Hundley, V.A., Cruickshank, F.M., Lang, G. et al. (1994). 'Midwife managed delivery unit: a randomised controlled comparison with consultant led care'. *British Medical Journal*, Vol. 309, pp. 1400–1404.

Hundley, V.A., Cruickshank, F.M., Milne, J.M. et al. (1995). 'Satisfaction and continuity of care: staff views of care in a midwife-managed delivery unit'. *Midwifery*, Vol. 11, pp. 163–173.

McCourt, C., Page, L. (Eds.) (1996). *Report on the Evaluation of One-to-One Midwifery.* London: Thames Valley University and The Hammersmith Hospital NHS Trust.

McIntosh, J. (1989). 'Models of childbirth and social class: a study of 80 working class primigravidae'. In: Robinson, S., Thomson, A. (Eds.) *Midwives Research and Childbirth. Vol. 1.* London: Chapman and Hall.

Rowley, M.J., Hensley, M.J., Brinamead, M.W., Wlodarczyk. (1995). 'Continuity of care by a midwife team versus routine care during pregnancy and birth: a randomised trial'. *Medical Journal of Australia,* Vol. 163, pp. 289–293.

Schott, J., Henley, A. (1996). *Culture, Religion and Childbearing: A Handbook for Health Professionals.* Oxford: Butterworth-Heinemann.

Sikorski, J., Wilson, J., Clement, S. et al. (1996). 'A randomised trial comparing two schedules of antenatal visits: the antenatal care project'. *British Medical Journal,* Vol. 312, pp. 546–53.

Tucker, J.S., Hall, M.H., Howie P.W. et al. (1996). 'Should obstetricians see women with normal pregnancies? A multicentre randomised controlled trial of routine antenatal care by general practitioners and midwives compared with shared care lead by obstetricians'. *British Medical Journal,* Vol. 312, pp. 554–59.

Turnbull, D., Holmes, A. et al. (1996). 'Randomised, controlled trial of efficacy of midwife-managed care'. *Lancet,* Vol. 348, pp. 213–218.

Twaddle, S., Liao, X.H., Fyvie, H. (1993). 'An evaluation of postnatal care individualised to the needs of the women'. *Midwifery,* Vol. 9, No. 3, pp. 154–160.

CHAPTER SIX

Assessing the Impact on Care Givers of Changes in Care

Jo Garcia, Rona Campbell, Jane Sandall, Trudy Stevens, Nancy MacKeith

This chapter is about longer-term issues like making change successfully, and setting up systems that will last. The sorts of questions that arise are: What can we learn about the process of change? How can others gain from our experience of setting up a new pattern of care? Are staff skills being used and developed in the new models of care? What are the advantages and disadvantages for staff of different ways of organizing care? Do the changes have an impact on the relations between different staff in maternity care? Perhaps the key question is 'How sustainable is a new pattern of care?'. Issues examined in studies of this area include individual responses to change, how the new system was introduced and whether the midwives in the new structures are self selected (Robinson, 1993; Warwick, 1995). There has been some very interesting work in this area as part of evaluations of changes in care (e.g. Currell, 1985; Hall et al., 1985; Hundley et al., 1995; Turnbull et al., 1995; McCourt and Page, 1996; Farquhar et al., 1996; Allen et al., 1997).

Background

During the 1960s and 70s maternity care became increasingly medicalized. The proportion of births taking place in institutions rose sharply from 64.4 per cent in 1957 to 98.5 per cent in 1979 as a result of policies which advocated phasing out home births on grounds of safety. The incidence of obstetric interventions, which first began to rise during the 1960s, also accelerated during the 1970s. The increasing medicalization of childbirth was accompanied by a fragmentation of maternity care. Antenatal care shared between the community and hospital was introduced because hospitals could no longer offer full antenatal care to the increasing numbers of women booked for delivery there. The organization of maternity care within hospitals also changed. Previously, postnatal wards had had several labour and delivery rooms attached and women were cared for by the same staff throughout their stay. With the introduction of centralized delivery suites, women were delivered by one set of staff and then passed on to another group for their postnatal care. Reductions in lengths of stay in hospital meant postnatal care being increasingly divided between hospital and home.

The involvement of general practitioners in maternity care also diminished during this period (Campbell and Macfarlane, 1994).

These changes were greeted with considerable concern by some user groups and by midwives who felt their role was being reduced from one of partnership with medicine to that of subservience. In 1983 the results of a national survey of midwives, obstetricians, general practitioners and health visitors, funded by the Department of Health and Social Security, showed that while midwives were responsible for providing much of the care, they were not able to exercise their clinical judgement as to how that care should be managed and delivered (Robinson, 1990). For example, it showed that less than five per cent of hospital midwives and one third of community midwives took sole responsibility for assessing the course of pregnancy. In most cases women were examined by medical staff after they had already been examined by midwives. It also demonstrated that midwives working in GP maternity units which were separate from consultant units were much more likely to have retained autonomy.

This important survey was an early example of research to assess the impact of change on care givers. Another contemporaneous national survey sought the views of mothers, midwives and obstetricians about intranatal care in general and induction in particular (Cartwright, 1979). Although this survey was focused on the active management of labour, it did contain some questions about the organization of care and in particular about home births. This showed that midwives over-estimated and obstetricians under-estimated the proportion of women who preferred home births. The proportions were 33 per cent (midwives), nine per cent (obstetricians) and 18 per cent (women). This finding highlights one of the difficulties in interpreting and acting on information on the views of care givers. Midwives are likely to exercise greater autonomy when delivering women at home and likewise obstetricians tend to control what happens in hospital. The views expressed may well be influenced by professional self interest.

In the 1980s new attitudes among care givers became more evident and there was a great deal of contact between user-groups, researchers and care givers. As the House of Commons Health Committee (1992) was reviewing the maternity services, discussions were taking place on practical measures designed to achieve more woman-centred care. A group of midwives came together to provide a framework in the face of little information and the need to avoid extra cost (Ball et al., 1991). This document and the book by Caroline Flint (1993) informed many midwifery managers as they worked out a system tailored to their unit, clients and midwives. Maternity services which had implemented schemes for midwifery-led care were often visited by midwives looking for ways to change their own units. Many publications have described the benefits and problems of new systems (Page, 1995; Lewis, 1995; Aston and Lee, 1995). Advocates of change emphasize the benefits for midwives of new models of care. Getting to know women well and having greater responsibility for their care is thought to be more satisfying for most midwives. New models of care can also provide opportunities for midwives to develop professionally, and to learn more about audit, and management of work.

There were anxieties, however, about the demands the new systems make on midwives' private lives and on the impact of the changes on the careers of midwives in different

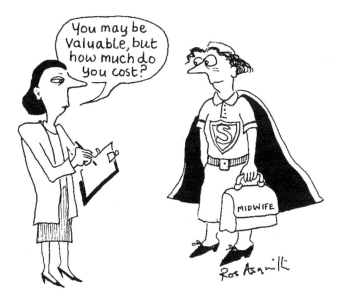

family circumstances (e.g. Stewart, 1995; Warwick, 1995; Sandall, 1995). Concern has also been expressed that women who voice their preferences in an articulate way may distract professional attention from those who are vulnerable because of poverty or isolation (Tyler, 1994). In addition, there is evidence that the changes in midwifery care were very diverse (Wraight et al., 1993) with some 'team' schemes having little potential to improve care for either women or midwives. Against this background midwives have also had to contend with the enormous upheaval brought about by the more general changes in the NHS. For example, their managers now quite frequently do not hold a midwifery qualification and, it is argued, do not therefore grasp the implications of a service for a basically healthy population. Recruitment and selection of midwives is an area with existing problems which need to be tackled as new systems of care come into place (MacKeith, 1994). When midwives from the previous culture of medically-led care 'select' future midwives to work in the new system will they be clear about the criteria which will be most useful in selection? Qualified clinical midwives and midwifery managers also need access to training and other resources in order to tackle changes in the organization of care.

The effect on other workers in the maternity services should not be underestimated. Obstetricians in maternity units have had varying degrees of involvement in discussions about the changes. Changes in the ways that wards are staffed by midwives are likely to have an impact on all grades of doctors, but particularly junior doctors and medical students. GPs are likely to be affected by changes in midwifery organization and are themselves undergoing various shifts in the way they work generally and in relation to maternity. Healthcare assistants are specifically included in the team midwifery framework from the Nuffield project (Ball et al., 1991). With fewer hospital midwives, the role of ancillary staff may become more important in hospital postnatal care. It is encouraging that some of the larger evaluations of new models of care are looking at the impact of changes in maternity organization on doctors and other non-midwifery staff (e.g. Hall et al., 1985; Green et al., 1994; Sikorski et al., 1995; Cheyne et al., 1995; Turnbull et al., 1995; Farquhar et al., 1996; Allen et al., 1997; Fleissig et al., 1997).

There are some specific problems with evaluating the effect of changes on care givers. Care givers may find this aspect of an evaluation particularly threatening. They may feel under pressure if their work is being observed or they may be reluctant to make their true views known, fearing that any adverse comments they make may rebound on them. Failure to take account of such concerns may compromise an evaluation, in an extreme case resulting in the withdrawal of co-operation of the care providers. Some of these concerns may be lessened if the person or people conducting the evaluation are completely independent from the organizations providing or purchasing care. Strong reassurances about anonymity in the way in which findings are reported should also help.

A problem of a different nature is how much weight should be given to the effect on staff when considering the findings of an evaluation. If the evaluation demonstrates unequivocally that a change in the organization of care has made intolerable demands on staff and that the new system is not sustainable, then even if users were very satisfied with the changes and the changes were found to be cost effective in the short term, clearly further change is going to be required. If, however, staff prefer the new system but users do not like it and there are no others differences in outcome, should the staff view be ignored? In the past, maternity services have tended to be organized according to what care providers, and in particular what obstetricians, thought best. The House of Commons Health Committee Report (1992) and *Changing Childbirth* have sought to redress that balance by stating that care should be woman centred.

Research approaches

There is a very wide range of appropriate research methods to be used in addressing the questions under this heading. Rather than going through all the alternatives we have chosen four studies to illustrate different approaches (see Boxes 6.1 and 6.2 and the two sections which follow them which have been written by co-authors of this chapter). The first study, reported in Box 6.1, describes a survey of midwifery staff which was undertaken prior to the introduction of changes in the service. The second study (see Box 6.2) involved a survey of all clinical staff in a large hospital maternity unit. This was undertaken to compliment data being collected in a randomized trial comparing shared care with midwifery led care. Unlike the first two studies, which depended on quantitative methods, an ethnographic approach was used by Trudy Stevens in the third study, to assess the impact of the introduction of 'One-to-One' midwifery on staff working in a London Trust. In the final study described here by Jane Sandall, a range of methods, both quantitative and qualitative, were used to study how the different ways of providing maternity care impacted on the working and personal lives of midwives. Useful references are listed at the end of the chapter.

Work of the kind that we have described here will be crucial in evaluating the various approaches to maternity care. It would be good if there were more studies to look at the views of GPs and obstetricians and at the ways that all the care-providers work together. If you are planning to study the views of staff at a local level, it is probably advisable to seek collaboration with independent researchers. This is because confidentiality is likely to be an issue; staff are more likely to take part, and to give their views freely, if they think that they will not be identified.

Box 6.1: Developing midwifery services in Swindon – using a self-administered questionnaire to look at the views of midwives in one centre prior to making changes in the service

This small study took place because midwifery managers in Swindon wanted to explore the views of midwifery staff before they implemented changes in the service. They also looked at women's views of care. The study was led by local research midwives who used a questionnaire which had been adapted to meet local midwifery practice from one developed at the National Perinatal Epidemiology Unit for the larger study on which this book was based (Garcia, 1997). That questionnaire was designed after pilot studies in three places, and using the experiences of other researchers.

The aims of the questionnaire were to:
a) describe the background, experience, home circumstances and current working pattern of midwives
b) assess their views about aspects of their work, and about new ways of working

Using a questionnaire like this provides only a static picture of what is happening to midwives, so it cannot help us to understand what changes are taking place. It does not deal with midwives who have left the service. It may also suffer from problems of lack of depth on some questions. In other words, respondents may tick a reply, but their views may not have been adequately allowed for in the options given, or may be too complex to express in a postal questionnaire.

The questionnaire was sent out from the hospital concerned but returned to the researchers at NPEU who had developed it. They carried out the analysis and provided the pooled results to the local research midwives. For reasons of confidentiality, care was taken in the way that data were presented in order to avoid the views of individuals being recognized. It was clear from the larger study that in some places midwives were very concerned that their individual views should not be identified by managers.

Results
Questionnaires were returned by 124 midwives out of 190 sent out (65%). A majority of respondents were clinical midwives working in the hospital.

The responses provided a detailed description of actual working patterns and views about issues like travel times, safety, shift lengths and on-call arrangements. Midwives were asked about their professional development and commented, for example, on whether their grade was appropriate for the work they were doing. They responded to quite a few questions about satisfaction with various aspects of the job and levels of stress and support. They were also asked about some features of their personal lives such as living situation and dependants in order to understand more about their commitments outside work. Many had young children, or other dependants. The midwives were asked about changes they would like to see and aspects of their system that they wanted to retain.

Their replies are being used to help plan changes in the service to address the recommendations in *Changing Childbirth* (Jones and Strong, 1996).

Box 6.2: Staff views of the Glasgow midwifery development unit – a study alongside a randomized controlled trial

The Midwifery Development Unit (MDU) was set up in the Glasgow Royal Maternity Hospital to provide and evaluate a programme of midwife-led care. The care was compared with shared care in a randomized controlled trial (Turnbull et al., 1996). The views of obstetricians and midwives were sought as part of the evaluation. In all 20 obstetricians and 85 midwives were surveyed using self-administered questionnaires. The questionnaire were made up of a number of short statements which the respondents were asked to respond to along a five point scale from 'strongly agree' to 'strongly disagree'. The obstetricians were studied in the course of the trial and the non-MDU midwives were surveyed before the system was set up and then during the trial. MDU midwives were studied before the system was set up and then regularly throughout the trial.

The obstetricians' survey was completed by 20 consultants and registrars working in the hospital. It was noted that on more than half the questions at least 25 per cent of respondents ticked 'not sure'. The authors wonder if this was due to a reluctance to pre-empt the results of the trial. The replies indicated that respondents were keen to remain involved in the care of low-risk women, though they recognized that the involvement of midwives could give them more time to devote to women at increased risk. There was some concern about liaison between MDU midwives and other care givers, particularly GPs. Respondents felt that midwives could provide appropriate care for low-risk women but that they needed a lot of support from obstetricians to do this (Cheyne et al., 1995).

The MDU midwives were different from the other midwives in various ways. They were slightly younger, more likely to be E-Grades and, before the scheme started, were more dissatisfied with their work. Their views of their work improved substantially during the course of the scheme. No comparable change was seen for non-MDU midwives over the same time period. There was no evidence of increased stress in MDU midwives in the 15 month period covered by the study. There were concerns expressed by midwives about some aspects of the setting up of the scheme and about liaison with colleagues. In this study, the questionnaire data collected regularly from MDU midwives was also used as feedback to those organising the scheme and changes were made as a result (Turnbull et al., 1995).

Tracing the ripples: an ethnographic study of the implementation of One-to-One midwifery practice

Trudy Stevens

Change is generally implemented in the belief that it will have positive benefits. However, people tend to react against change and, in so doing, may negatively influence the change process. Also, the change implemented may have ramifications that affect the service in unexpected ways. Acknowledging this, an ethnographic study was included in the evaluation of a radical service change implemented by the Centre for Midwifery Practice, within the Hammersmith Hospitals' NHS Trust.

Embodying the recommendations of *Changing Childbirth*, One-to-One Midwifery Practice was introduced within the Trust in November 1993. Twenty midwives were organized in partnerships within three group practices. Each carried a caseload of 40 high and low risk women per year. Offering midwifery-led, GP-led, or obstetric-led care, the midwives provided antenatal, intrapartum and postnatal care in the community or in the hospital as required.

An extensive evaluation of this innovative service was planned, using a comparative design based on the local postal districts. The study focused on four different dimensions, using both quantitative and qualitative research methods. It included:

- a study of the effect on consumers using a longitudinal, self-completion questionnaire and both individual and focus group interviews;
- an assessment of standards of care and adherence to targets using clinical audit;
- an evaluation of resource use through an economic audit; and
- documentation and analysis of the process of change, using an ethnographic approach, with a particular focus on the implications for staff.

Details of the complete study can be found elsewhere (McCourt and Page, 1996). This account is purely concerned with the quantitative work.

Why ethnography?

Ethnography is a research approach which seeks primarily to describe and understand a social situation and its meaning for those involved, rather than to measure outcomes. It is particularly useful in studies of organizations, where individuals' interpretations of their environment and of their own and others' behaviour is important. A particular strength of this approach is the ability to highlight the different perspectives of individuals, frequently uncovering the views of the less powerful, and to explore whether issues hold different significance for different people. In studies of change it can help by identifying misperceptions and problem areas which, when appreciated, may then be addressed.

Recognizing that what people say and what they do may differ, and that interviews can be unduly influenced by particular events, data are collected by a variety of means, from a variety of sources, over a prolonged period of time. This 'triangulation' of data collection helps to avoid biases, and to paint a detailed picture of what is going on. The aim of the approach is to explore and understand a social situation, and to be open to the unexpected. Thus, it is important that the researcher does not impose any preconceived ideas on the study, and that the data themselves dictate the subsequent analysis, although for evaluative purposes particular questions may need to be addressed, e.g. 'will midwives work this way?'; 'what preparation did they find helpful?'; 'what were obstetricians' initial, and subsequent, concerns?' (see Baillie, 1995 for a succinct critique of ethnography and nursing research).

My appointment as a social scientist and midwife from outside the One-to-One scheme helped reassure respondents that their views would be respected and anonymity maintained. My familiarity with maternity services helped me establish easy relationships with the staff and to approach them appropriately. By living on-site during the week, I have been able to collect data at times and in circumstances that are best suited to a 24 hours service; chats during meals in the canteen, unexpected meetings in the corridor, and evening visits to the wards and delivery unit have proved particularly helpful in developing people's trust, gaining their views and developing an understanding of what is going on. Issues raised at these times are tested and explored further during subsequent formal data collection procedures such as interviews.

More formal data collection has been undertaken by:

- individual interviews and focus group meetings;
- participant observation of relevant managers', midwives' and project meetings;
- documentary analysis of papers generated, and the minutes of meetings held during the planning and implementation period prior to my appointment.

Informed by the preliminary analysis, participant observation of staff interactions within the clinical setting may be undertaken during a later stage of the study.

Individual interviews with all people possibly affected by change would have generated an overwhelming amount of data and demanded enormous resources of time. A mixture of individual and focus-group interviews was undertaken in order to gain a broad range of perspectives, establishing a balance between the ideal and the practical.

Specific people targeted for interview have been:

- key individuals (e.g. clinical director, project leader);
- members of key groups, where the number was small (e.g. One-to-One midwives, managers, different grades of obstetrician, senior hospital midwives);
- midwives leaving the Trust (One-to-One and hospital).

Focus-group work has been undertaken with larger groups such as midwives working in specific areas – community, clinic, hospital wards and delivery unit – and with student midwives.

The danger of becoming so absorbed into the organizational culture so as to be unable to view it objectively ('going native') is partly overcome by weekends away from the hospital; this enabled me to stand back and become the 'outsider' once more.

Appropriate supervision and participation in academic and professional seminars has also proved helpful in questioning my assumptions and raising new issues for investigation.

The findings from studies such as this one are very context specific; people's perceptions are unique to particular situations – they cannot be generalized to other populations. Nevertheless, many of the issues raised may be applicable elsewhere and so the findings can serve to sensitize others following a similar change process. This study is continuing, tracing the pattern of changes over time. However, some of the themes emerging from the preliminary analyses conducted to meet the needs of the evaluation (McCourt and Page, 1996) are presented here to illustrate the sort of issues this approach can highlight.

Implementing the change

This required enormous energy on the part of the implementation team and the planning phase was much longer than expected; a shared vision and common goal appeared to be of paramount importance during this period. However, despite very careful planning, unexpected developments within the wider organization seriously affected the implementation. It is easy to forget that the context of change is change, that life and social situations are not static; thus the movement to Trust status, a new Chief Executive, new Clinical Director and new Head of Midwifery all had important implications for the project. Effective, *on-going* communication at all levels proved essential and the value of informal communication strategies was highlighted.

Some midwives really enjoy working this way. Recruited from within the Trust, the majority were not very experienced (minimum one year post-registration), but all were strongly motivated towards woman-centred care and strongly dissatisfied with working within the conventional service. It took about nine months for them to settle into the new way of working, and the development of time-management and organizational skills proved crucial. During this time the attitude of the midwifery managers, and their movement between supervisor and manager roles, was central in supporting midwives adapting to the changes; an enabling rather than controlling management style appeared fundamental.

Midwives report appreciating the flexibility and autonomy of this style of work and gaining intense satisfaction from the different relationships formed with women and their families, and with professional colleagues. Once midwives were used to this style of work, problem areas mainly related to having to work (and travel) between two very different hospitals, and the interface with the conventional hospital service. This latter problem was also highlighted by the hospital-based midwives who perceived the One-to-One midwives as elitist and, at times, not pulling their weight. The development of the new service was seen to imply a devaluation of the service and hard work of both hospital and community midwives – a perception which could be mitigated if the development of an innovation were accompanied by support and development of the staff not directly involved.

Student midwives acknowledged the restrictions placed on their social lives, but reported that the continuity of care provides a real learning experience, enabling them to assess their advice and treatment. However, having been trained within a *Changing Childbirth* curriculum and experienced working that way, many expressed extreme reluctance to work in the conventional system; a situation that may have important ramifications for recruitment.

Obstetric staff at all levels expressed support for the development although several were concerned as to whether midwives were willing or able to work this way. Their subsequent experience indicated a positive impact of caseload midwifery, particularly on the provision of antenatal care. However, tensions arose on delivery unit, where obstetricians of all levels felt excluded from the One-to-One deliveries. Without the routine 'social visit' of the 'round' at change of duty, they suggested that if they were called into a problem situation late in labour, they might be forced to practice 'rescue obstetrics' on women they had never met.

Ethnography as aid for change

As part of an evaluation rather than pure research, the study sought to help solve problems rather than just gain knowledge. Close interaction between members of the research and implementation teams helped inform the project development. However, the maintenance of confidentiality was paramount at all times: issues commonly raised were fed back to the team in a general way; in specific situations, individuals were encouraged to take their problems to the appropriate people.

Some people appeared to really appreciate being given the opportunity to talk about the issues that concerned them; interviews are not only a demonstration that people's opinions are valued, but the process of being encouraged to formulate and discuss what may only be vague feelings can be beneficial.

In conclusion, most qualitative studies may be helpful in assessing staff reactions and, by giving people an alternative channel through which to express their concerns and a process of feedback, may actually assist with the change process.

Changing Childbirth: the impact on midwives and midwifery work

Jane Sandall

This project was still in progress as the book was being compiled (funded by the NHS Executive Doctoral Research Training Scheme). The aims were:

- To examine the impact of changing occupational roles and responsibilities on midwives' practice and their experience of work.
- To examine the impact of providing continuity of care for midwives' personal lives in terms of personal accomplishment and burnout.

Exploratory case study

Stage 1 of the study, carried out in 1994–5, was an exploratory case study in three sites. It aimed to identify the organizational, professional and personal factors that contribute to the successes and failures of different approaches to providing a woman-centred model of care. Sites were chosen to represent variations in the organization and provision of continuity of midwifery care. The sites were:

1.   The self-managed group practice – one to one continuity. This was an urban group practice of self-employed midwives who each had a personal caseload of 34 'high and low' risk women.

2.   The traditional model – antenatal and postnatal continuity. This site involved GP attached community midwives in a semi-rural area who provided continuity of care in the antenatal and postnatal period to a caseload of 137 mainly low risk women and delivered about 10 per cent of their caseload personally.

3.   The team model – team continuity. Three urban community-based teams were studied. They were within the NHS and shared a team caseload of 216 'high and low' risk women, plus the postnatal care of 100 women who delivered in other units.

Field work of four to six weeks in each site consisted of observation of midwifery work and the collection of policy and audit documents. Tape recorded semi-structured interviews of about one to two hours were carried out with a sample of midwives (N = 48) and key informants. Topics covered in the interview included the following:

- biographical and attitudinal data;
- roles and responsibilities and organization of work;
- orientation to midwifery;
- decision making and practice style;
- job satisfaction and stress;
- collegial relationships;
- relationships with mothers.

The qualitative data generated were transcribed and analysed using Hyper Research, a computerized qualitative data analysis package and will be integrated with the survey data. Interviews with 48 midwives along with observation of organizational and clinical practice generated three key factors relating to sustainable caseload midwifery, the avoidance of burnout and the provision of woman centred care (Sandall, 1997). These were:

- occupational autonomy
- emotional and social support at home and work
- developing meaningful relationships with women.

All the midwives in the self-managed practice and a few of the GP attached midwives had personal caseloads. These midwives had increased control over how they organized their work and were more able to develop meaningful relationships with women due to greater continuity of carer. Because of the increased control, they were more able to integrate family responsibilities with their work and to respond flexibly to women's needs. These two factors also influenced their experience of being on-call which was less stressful and easier to integrate into their personal life than midwives with a team caseload. Conversely, midwives with a team caseload had less control over how they organized their work and were not able to get to 'know' women as well. Midwives were able to combine caseload midwifery with childcare commitments provided they had control and flexibility over how they organized their work and had social and emotional support networks at home and work.

Overall, control and continuity are as important to midwives in how well they balance their work and home life as they are to women experiencing childbirth. The way that midwifery work is organized can either increase or decrease the likelihood of burnout, and models of care that incorporate these factors are more likely to be sustainable and to provide more flexible woman centred care.

Survey of practising midwives

The second stage of the research was carried out during 1995 and provided an overview of the current organization of midwives' work in England. Approximately 90 per cent of all practising midwives in England and Wales belong to the RCM, and in England 22,975 midwives were full members. A postal questionnaire was sent to a geographically stratified five per cent sample of the membership of the Royal College of Midwives; 1166 midwives were surveyed and a response rate of 69 per cent was achieved. This sampling frame provided a representative picture of midwives in England and was large enough to enable comparisons to be made between particular categories.

The questionnaire used in the survey was developed during the first stage of the study and piloted on a small sample of midwives. The questionnaire included:

- biographical details;
- organization of work;
- occupational autonomy;
- job satisfaction, stress and burnout;
- attitudes of midwives to 'woman-centred care';
- how midwives with domestic responsibilities manage their working life.

Occupational burnout was measured with the Maslach Burnout Inventory (Maslach and Jackson, 1986) and psychological distress measured using the General Health Questionnaire – GHQ-12 (Goldberg 1992). Both these instruments have been used for similar purposes in this country and abroad. The analysis of the survey data focused on three key issues: the relationship between the organization of midwifery work and occupational autonomy; the experiences of midwives who were working mothers; and factors at home and work that were related to high burnout rates.

The psychometric properties of the stress inventories were tested for validity and reliability in the qualitative and quantitative part of the project. Factors at work and in the home were identified that were significantly associated with higher burnout scores;

midwives with low control over their work pattern and decison making, those who worked full time and those who spent the longest time travelling to work were more likely to suffer burnout. Domestic and child-care responsibilities had no impact on burnout once other factors were controlled for in the analysis. Further details of these findings will be reported in due course.

References

Allen, I., Bourke Dowling, S., Williams, S. (1997). *A Leading Role for Midwives*. London: Policy Studies Institute.

Aston, G., Lee, B. (1995). 'Moving forward on the Cumberledge Report – Changing Childbirth'. *Journal of the the Royal Society of Medicine,* Vol. 88, pp. 115–118.

Baillie, L. (1995). 'Ethnography and nursing research: a critical appraisal'. *Nurse Researcher,* Vol. 3, No. 2, pp. 5–21.

Ball. J., Flint, C., Garvey, M., Jackson-Baker, A., Page, L. (1991). *Who's Left Holding the Baby? An Organisational Framework for Making the Most of Midwifery Services.* Leeds: Nuffield Institute for Health Services Studies.

Campbell. R., Macfarlane, A. (1994). *Where to be Born? The Debate and the Evidence.* Oxford: National Perinatal Epidemiology Unit.

Cartwright, A. (1979). *The Dignity of Labour?* Tavistock: London.

Cheyne, H., Turnbull, D., Lunan, C.B., Reid, M., Greer, I.A. (1995). 'Working alongside a midwife-led unit: what do obstetricians think?'. *British Journal of Obstetrics and Gynaecology,* Vol. 102, pp. 485–487.

Currell, R. (1985). *Continuity and Fragmentation in Maternity Care.* Unpublished MPhil dissertation, University of Exeter.

Farquhar, M., Camilleri-Ferrante, C., Todd, C. (1996). *An Evaluation of Midwifery Teams in West Essex – Executive Summary.* Cambridge: Cambridge University Institute of Public Health.

Fleissig, A., Kroll, D., McCarthy, M. (1997). 'General practitioners' views on the implementation of community-led maternity care in South Camden, London'. *British Journal of General Practice,* Vol. 47, pp. 45–46.

Flint, C. (1993). *Midwifery Teams and Caseloads.* London: Butterworth-Heinemann.

Garcia, J. (1997). *Changing Midwifery Care – The Scope for Evaluation Report of an NHSE-Funded Project.* Oxford: National Perinatal Epidemiology Unit.

Goldberg, D. (1992). *The General Health Questionnaire.* NFER-NELSON

Green, J., Kitzinger, J., Coupland, V. (1994). 'Midwives' responsibilities, medical staffing structures and women's choices in childbirth'. In: Robinson, S., Thomson, A. (Eds). *Midwives, Research and Childbirth, Vol 3.* London: Chapman and Hall.

Hall, M., Macintyre, S., Porter, M. (1985). *Antenatal Care Assessed.* Aberdeen: Aberdeen University Press.

House of Commons Health Committee (1992). *Maternity Services.* London: HMSO.

Hundley, V., Cruikshank, F.M., Milne, J.M., Glazener, C.M.A., Lang, G.D., Turner, M., Blyth, D., Mollinson, J. (1995). 'Satisfaction and continuity of care: staff views of care in a midwife-managed delivery unit'. *Midwifery,* Vol. 11, pp. 163–173.

Jones, J., Strong, P. (1996). *Developing Midwifery Services: Report on Results of the Questionnaire for Midwives.* Princess Margaret Hospital, Swindon.

Lewis, P. (1995). 'Developing a group practice approach to care'. *MIDIRS Midwifery Digest,* Vol. 5, pp. 104–8.

McCourt, C., Page, L. (Eds.) (1996). *Report on the Evaluation of One-to-One Midwifery Practice The Centre for Midwifery Practice.* London: The Hammersmith Hospitals NHS and Thames Valley University.

MacKeith, N. (1994). *Delivering the Pre-registration Midwifery Student: Recruitment and Selection for Pre-Registration Midwifery in England.* Unpublished Dissertation.

Maslach, C., Jackson, S.E. (1986). *Maslach Burnout Inventory.* Palo Alto, California: Consulting Psychologists Press.

Page, L. (1995). *Effective Group Practice in Midwifery.* Oxford: Blackwell Science.

Robinson, S. (1990). 'Maintaining the independence of the midwifery profession: a continuing struggle'. In: Garcia, J., Kilpatrick, R., Richards, M. (Eds). *The Politics of Maternity Care.* Oxford: Oxford University Press.

Robinson, S. (1993). 'Combining work with caring for children; findings from a longitudinal study'. *Midwifery,* Vol. 9, pp. 183–196.

Sandall, J. (1995). 'Choice, continuity and control: changing midwifery – towards a sociological perspective'. *Midwifery,* Vol. 11, pp. 201–9.

Sandall, J. (1997). 'Midwives' burnout and continuity of care'. *British Journal of Midwifery,* Vol. 5, No. 2, pp. 106–111.

Sikorski, J., Clement, S., Wilson, J., Das, S., Smeeton, N. (1995). 'A survey of health professionals' views on possible changes in the provision and organisation of antenatal care'. *Midwifery,* Vol. 11, pp. 61–68.

Stewart, M. (1995). 'Do you have to know your midwife?'. *British Journal of Midwifery,* Vol. 3, pp. 19–20.

Turnbull, D., Reid, M., McGinley, M., Sheilds, N. (1995). 'Changes in midwives' attitudes to their professional role following the implementation of the midwifery development unit'. *Midwifery,* Vol. 11, pp. 110–119.

Turnbull, D., Holmes, A., Sheilds, N., Cheyne, H. et al. (1996). 'Randomised controlled trial of efficacy of midwife-managed care', *Lancet,* Vol. 348, pp. 213–218.

Tyler, S. (1994). 'Maternity care and the paradox of plenty'. *British Journal of Midwifery,* Vol. 2, pp. 552–554.

Warwick, C. (1995). 'Midwives and maternity leave' *Maternity Action,* Vol. 67, pp. 6–7.

Wraight, A., Ball, J., Seccombe, I., Stock, J. (1993). *Mapping Team Midwifery.* IMS Report No. 242. Brighton: Institute of Manpower Studies.

Further reading

Ethnography and phenomenology *Nurse Researcher* Vol. 3, No. 2, 1995.

Observation *Nurse Researcher* Vol. 2, No. 2, 1994.

Action Research *Nurse Researcher* Vol. 2, No. 3, 1995.

Bakker, R.H.C., Groenewegen, P.P., Jabaaij, L., Meijer, W., Sixma, H., deVeer, A. (1997). '"Burnout" among Dutch midwives'. *Midwifery,* Vol. 12, pp. 174–181.

Ball, J.A., Washbrook, M. (1996). *Birthrate Plus: A Framework for Workforce Planning and Decision-making for Midwifery Services.* Hale, Cheshire: Books for Midwives Press.

Dopson, S., Waddington, I. (1996). 'Managing social change: a process-sociological approach to understanding organisational change within the National Health Service'. *Sociology of Health and Illness,* Vol. 18, pp. 525–550.

Hammersley, M., Atkinson, P. (1995). *Ethnography: Principles in Practice.* 2nd edition. London: Routledge.

Hunt, S., Symonds, A. (1995). *The Social Meaning of Midwifery.* London: Macmillan.

Lathlean, J. (1994). 'Choosing an appropriate methodology'. In: Buckledee, J., McMahon, R. (Eds). *The Research Experience in Nursing.* London: Chapman and Hall.

Lofland, J., Lofland, L.H. (1984). *Analyzing Social Settings: A Guide to Qualitative Observation and Analysis.* 2nd edition. California: Wadsworth Publishing Company.

Stock, J., Wraight, A. (1993). *Developing Continuity of Care in Maternity Services; The Implications for Midwives.* Report to the Royal College of Midwives. Brighton: Institute of Manpower Studies.

Yin, R.K. (1989). *Case Study Research: Design and Methods. Applied Social Research Methods Series.* Volume 5. London: Sage.

CHAPTER SEVEN

Economic Evaluation

James Piercy and Miranda Mugford

Whenever the phrase 'economic evaluation' is mentioned, one of the first things that is thought about is money. Equally, whenever 'change' is suggested, probably the first thought which crosses the mind of health service staff, and of managers in particular, is how much the change will cost.

As has been discussed earlier in this book, evaluation means finding out if something is of value. The results of an economic evaluation may indicate what the benefits and costs are as a result of an intervention. However, the purpose of economic evaluation should only be as an input to decision making. Although there is no magic formula for translating the results of evaluation into policy, economists have some tools for describing benefits in economic terms which will tell a decision maker whether the benefit is worth the cost which would be incurred. This decision is left with the manager and stakeholder concerned, even though the evaluation will inform this decision.

Whenever there is any change in the method of service delivery, there will be some implication for resource use. In many cases, there will be trade-offs between resources, often between different sectors, such as hospital and community. Economics offers a methodology for analysing these questions, and is an important component in an increasing number of evaluations. Some examples of recently published economic evaluations in maternity care are given in Box 7.1.

The remainder of this chapter focuses on key issues regarding:

- the types and nature of economic evaluation;
- costs;
- benefits;
- information sources, methods of resource use data collection and data analysis;
- combining costs and benefits;
- preparation of reports;
- further reading.

Box 7.1: Economic aspects of alternative patterns of antenatal care: The Scottish antenatal care trial and team midwifery care in Birmingham

Scottish antenatal care trial

A multicentre randomized trial has recently been reported which compared different approaches to providing antenatal care for 'low risk' women in Scotland. The comparison was between shared care, then the routine form of care in Scotland, in which much care is given by hospital obstetric and midwifery staff, and care led by GPs and community midwives. The trial was designed to answer economic questions, in addition to the question of clinical effectiveness. The study was designed to measure the costs of care received by women in either form of care, and the costs to women of travel and waiting, and to estimate the preferences that women attached to the care they received, using survey methods to estimate 'willingness to pay'. The results of the trial showed that there was no difference in key measures of clinical effectiveness, that the community based programme of care resulted in lower costs per woman, and that there was no significant difference in the women's willingness to pay for the alternative forms of care (Tucker et al., 1996; Ratcliffe, Ryan and Tucker, 1996; Ryan, Ratcliffe and Tucker; 1997).

Team midwifery care in Birmingham

The Health Service Management centre in Birmingham has recently undertaken an evaluation of a new pattern of maternity care, designed to offer services in accordance with the objectives of *Changing Childbirth*. The subject of the evaluation was a team midwifery pilot scheme providing care for 24 hours a day, seven days a week. Midwives in the scheme worked in both hospital and community setting, with the intention of offering continuity of carer throughout the childbearing period. The study was designed to investigate not only economic issues but also women's experiences of care. Women in the pilot group experienced increased overall levels of satisfaction and reported enhanced choice and continuity of carer. No significant differences in clinical outcomes were observed, but the study was not designed to show such changes. It was found that the midwifery and associated costs such as travel and telephones were higher in the pilot group. However it was recognized that if the scheme was to be extended to include more women, then there could well be some cost reductions as a result of economies of scale. Of particular importance was the shorter length of stay in the pilot group. Were the scheme to be extended to include more women, the reduction in required bed days could be sufficient to lead to significant cost savings, which would offset at least some of the extra costs of the team midwives (Health Services Management Centre and Birmingham Women's Health Care Trust (1996). *Woman-focused Care – At What Cost? A Resource Manual.* Enquiries to: Midwifery Administration, Birmingham Women's Health Care NHS Trust, Birmingham B15 2TG)

Who is interested in the results of economic evaluation?

Many people are interested in the results of economic evaluation, both at a local and a national level. Clearly, the level of interest will depend on the nature of the project being evaluated. Minor changes will have only local interest; major service changes or developments, particularly if innovations such as 'one-to-one' or caseload midwifery are involved, will arouse national interest. Reports will be of particular interest when there are general lessons to learn and ideas to share. All evaluations, however small, will have local value. Interested parties may well include:

- midwifery managers;
- business managers;
- clinical directors;
- local service purchasers;
- GPs;
- local consumer groups.

Some evaluations, typically large-scale and far-reaching or those involving service innovations will have a general interest, as well as local interest. Clearly, it is not sensible to evaluate every scheme in every hospital, so findings need to be disseminated. Often it is a condition of the body awarding funding that results are shared through publications, workshops and presentations. Small evaluations, particularly those funded in-house, are not subject to such requirements; wider dissemination will be at the discretion of the researcher and the Trust. Note, however, that confidential information relating to patients (and also hospital finances) should not be distributed; results should be written up in more general terms. The potential degree of interest will determine the scale and perhaps the method of evaluation, though all evaluations (of course) should be done as rigorously as possible given the key input to decision making. The presentation of the results is also likely to be different.

What is economic evaluation?

Definition of economic evaluation

Economic evaluation aims to identify, measure, value and compare the costs and outcomes, or consequences, of alternative courses of action. The scope of analysis is related to the perspective chosen. Is the evaluator looking solely at health service implications or are women's costs going to be considered? The depth of the analysis relates to the extent to which detailed patient data will be collected, and thus to how precise the estimates of resource-use will be. However, if these data are not routinely available, then information requirements will be large. If no data are available, then economic evaluation can take the form of a modelling exercise, using estimates of resource use and outcome from sources such as the literature and professional judgement. This type of evaluation is more complicated and requires extensive sensitivity analysis where results are calculated for a range of different assumptions or cost values. Economic evaluations without data (i.e. modelling exercises) are not for the faint hearted!

Characteristics of economic evaluation

There are three key characteristics which will be present in any type of economic evaluation, regardless of the scale of the evaluation or to whom the results will be of interest or value. The first characteristic is that economic evaluation should be *undertaken prospectively,* that is before the actual decision is made. Remember that the purpose of economic evaluation is as an aid to decision making. The evaluation can be either hypothetical – where the costs and benefits of the action are estimated and modelled – or can involve a study. This allows the costs and benefits of the intervention or action to be directly estimated (Sculpher et al., 1997).

Secondly, in economic evaluation, there must be a *choice of at least two alternatives.* Evaluation is comparative; usually the new alternative is considered and compared to a baseline, typically the existing situation *before* making changes or to a control group at the same time period. For example, an evaluation of a new system of midwifery organization would be compared against the existing or prior situation.

Thirdly, an evaluation must consider *both the costs and the benefits* of the introduction of a new treatment or care scheme. It is not enough simply to look at the costs of a scheme and ignore the benefits, or to evaluate benefits without considering the costs. Indeed, it is the way in which costs and benefits are measured which determines which type of evaluation is appropriate.

Types of economic evaluation

There are two principal types of economic evaluation: cost-benefit analysis (CBA) and cost-effectiveness analysis (CEA). The key differences between them are set out in the following table, in terms of how the costs and benefits are measured, and what the appropriate decision rules are.

	COST-BENEFIT	**COST-EFFECTIVENESS**
Measurement of costs & benefits	Same units	Different units
Measurement of costs	Money	Money
Measurement of benefits	Money	a. Natural units e.g. cases detected in a screening programme b. Utility e.g. life years gained c. Other outcomes*
Decision rule	Accept Option A if benefits of A exceed the costs of A	Accept Option A if the relative benefits of B to A are not worth the additional costs of B relative to A

* can be any outcome as long as it can be measured and compared

Table 7.1: Characteristics of economic evaluation

The 'decision rule' relates to the question of whether an intervention or change will be accepted and implemented. It is the way in which costs and benefits are measured that influences the decision rule.

Which type of study is appropriate?

This depends on the question to be addressed. If the question is simply, is Option A worth doing at all, then the decision rule is basically whether the benefits of A exceed the costs, and CBA is used. Alternatively, and this is more common, if the question asked is whether Option A is better than Option B, then either CBA or CEA can be used, depending on how benefits are measured. If benefits can be calculated in money terms, use CBA, if they cannot be then CEA is appropriate. For decisions about the organization of midwifery practice, it is likely that CEA would be used. Note that in CEA, the costs of the alternatives still need to be considered, and this will provide an answer to the question of whether a new alternative is affordable or not.

The question for consideration

Before launching into a discussion of costs and benefits, it is crucial for the researcher to understand exactly what question they are addressing and from what perspective. This will help the researcher decide what to analyse, what type of study to use and what data to collect.

A good starting point is to state an hypothesis which can be tested. Hypotheses make statements about the relationship between variables, and allow a researcher to devise a method of testing them. For example, an hypothesis may be 'Does continuity of carer reduce the need for hospital admission?'. As well as setting the question, the hypothesis also dictates which data need to be collected. The research question gives a structure for the study. Once this has been done, the next stage is to identify which data need to be collected. Economic appraisal requires collection of both cost and outcome (or consequence/effectiveness) data. The following sections consider what is meant by 'cost' and how to interpret cost figures, benefits, and (importantly) data sources.

Costs

As mentioned in the previous section, economic analysis and evaluation always involve costs. What are costs, and how do costs change as the pattern of care (and therefore resource consumption) changes? The aim of this section is to explain what costs are, how NHS costs are identified and presented, the link between changing resource utilization and changing costs, and what costs need to be taken into consideration in economic evaluation.

What is a cost?

Costs are a measure of what has to be given up in order to achieve something. Typically, in the NHS, the cost would be defined as the amount of money which would need to be spent – the outlay. This is an accounting definition: economists would measure cost in terms of the alternative use of the resource – what has to be foregone in order to achieve the particular outcome or objective. An example illustrating these two concepts concerns the cost of a community antenatal visit by a midwife. An accountant would measure the cost as being the value of the midwife's time plus travel expenses and any consumables used for tests and so on. An economist would measure the cost in terms of the value of an activity which has to be foregone in order to undertake the antenatal visit, for example, the number of out-patient attendances by other women to see that midwife in the same space of time. The two definitions coincide if the prices with which the outlay is calculated reflect the value of the alternative use of the resource.

Costs in the NHS reflect the money value of the resource used; and to undertake economic evaluation, prices need to be attached to each resource used in the delivery of care. The remainder of this chapter explains how costs might be obtained and how they might be used in evaluation.

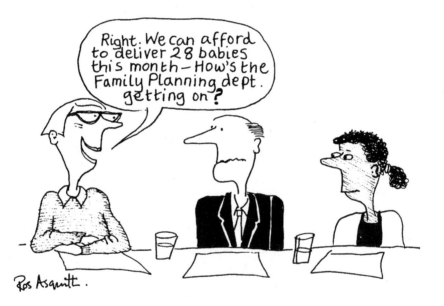

Basic definitions

Before going on to explain how costs in the NHS are presented, and how they might be used, it is necessary to outline a few basic concepts and definitions. These are explained in Boxes 7.2 and 7.3 and have been kept to a minimum.

Box 7.2: Direct, indirect and overhead costs – accountancy terminology

These terms relate to the way in which costs can be broken down and attributed to particular activities, such as ward costs, theatre costs, community midwifery and diagnostic testing. With respect to the costing component of evaluation, it is vital to be aware of direct, indirect and overhead costs, if only to ensure that nothing is left out. For example, the costing of ultrasound scanning cannot be undertaken without considering the cost of the scanner itself, even though it may be used for activities other than maternity care. This is particularly important when considering ward costs.

DIRECT costs are those which can be attributed directly to a particular activity or cost centre. For example, the amount of dressings and drugs consumed by a ward or department can be directly attributed to it through hospital information systems. This is done automatically by finance departments. Drugs and dressings are therefore direct costs of the ward (or theatre, patient or procedure).

INDIRECT costs are those costs which cannot be attributed directly to a particular cost centre, but can be shared across a number of them. These costs can then be apportioned to a particular department or ward. Medical staffing is one such cost, given that doctors will typically have responsibility for gynaecology as well as for maternity care. Equally, within maternity, medical staff costs would need to be apportioned between wards, out-patients and any other activities.

OVERHEAD costs are the costs of general and support services which contribute to the general running of a hospital, but cannot directly be related to any ward or activity. These might include planning, finance and general maintenance.

To give a practical example of this type of cost classification, consider a family of four drivers who have the use of one car which they keep in a large garage. The cost of petrol is a direct cost, since this can be attributed directly to each driver because it is known how much they use (approximately). The costs of servicing, tax and insurance are indirect costs; they are all concerned with the car, but not directly attributable to each driver. These costs can, of course, be apportioned, for example, in relation to usage. The cost of maintaining the garage is an overhead cost, since the garage is (could also be) used to store bicycles, coal, the fridge freezer, garden tools etc., not just for keeping the car.

The above definitions have been taken from NHS Executive guidance. However, in conducting evaluations, researchers should discuss with finance staff or take external advice from economists unless they are confident that they can derive sensible cost estimates themselves. The purpose of including the above definitions is to make researchers aware of the nature of costs and of some of the basic terminology. Economists use the term 'indirect costs' to refer to costs arising externally to health care: changes in the earning power of patients as a result of different treatments, for example. It is a good idea to check what definition has been used when you are reading a cost study.

Box 7.3: Fixed, semi-fixed and variable costs – economic costing

---

In terms of economic evaluation, this breakdown of total cost is far more useful since it relates to how costs actually change as activity changes. All new developments will involve some change in activity and therefore some change in resource use. Assessment of the effects on costs of changes in activity is crucial to understanding an economic evaluation. Brief definitions of this type of cost are outlined next:

VARIABLE costs are those costs which will vary with any change in activity. Hence, changes in activity will have a direct effect on cost. Examples of variable costs include disposable equipment, drugs, chemicals and dressings.

FIXED costs are those costs which are unaffected by short run changes in activity. Clearly in the long run, all costs can be varied, but for the purpose of most midwifery evaluations, many costs are fixed. Examples of fixed costs include general management, senior nursing and medical staff and maintenance. To highlight the distinction between fixed and variable costs, consider your telephone bill. The standing charge or line rental is a fixed cost, since it does not vary regardless of the number of calls made or received. The call charge is a variable cost, since it varies directly with the number of telephone calls made.

One further category is important, and that is semi-fixed costs. These are crucial to understand, since they account for over half of total NHS expenditure.

SEMI-FIXED costs are those costs which are fixed over a given range of activity, but may increase or fall as activity rises or drops below specific levels. Nursing and midwifery costs are a good example of semi-fixed costs. Consider, as an example, a ward with 24 beds. If the number of beds was to be reduced by one, say, it would be unlikely that a reduction in ward midwifery staff would follow. Equally, if two beds were removed, there would be little or no impact on staff numbers on any one shift. If, however, twelve beds were closed, then there may be scope for reducing the number of midwives per shift. At some point between closing two or twelve beds, it might be possible to staff the ward safely with one fewer midwife per shift. However, without having more information about the ward, it is hard to say where and at what point this reduction in staff would occur. That particular point is known as a 'step', and represents a sufficiently large change in activity for semi-fixed costs to change. To identify that point the researcher would need to hold discussions with midwifery staff and managers – professional judgement may need to be used.

Identifying which costs are classed as direct, indirect and overhead, or fixed, semi-fixed and variable does not always appear to be a straightforward task. However, there are clear rules laid out to assist with this process. The NHS Executive has stated for all types of costs the precise category into which they fall for accountancy purposes. This is published in 'Costing for Contracting', a copy of which should be held in hospital finance departments.

Resources or costs?

When undertaking evaluation, and before costing can take place, the resource implications of a change in service delivery have to be identified. Indicators of the use of health service resources that may need to be measured could include one or more of the following:

- number of admissions;
- length of hospital stay;
- number of out-patient attendances;
- antenatal and postnatal contacts;
- method of delivery and use of facilities;
- tests and investigations;
- drugs, including pain relief.

The differences between resources and costs are outlined in Box 7.4.

Box 7.4: Costs and resource use

- Resources are the staff, equipment, buildings and materials required to provide care.
- Costs are the money value of these resources.

In an evaluation of continuous support during labour, Mugford (1996) found that resources required were +92.5 hours of additional midwifery time per 100 women and -14.75 hours per 100 women of medical time. The actual cost change depends on whether there is additional midwifery time available (opportunity cost of zero) and whether medical time would be freed for other uses.

Any contact between the woman and the NHS will use resources. However, researchers only need to collect data which are relevant to the evaluation question. For example, in a study concerning the organization of community midwives, data relating to women booked entirely for hospital care may not be relevant if their care does not change as a result of the policy. There is no advantage in collecting data on resource use which is unlikely to change as a result of the proposed change in the service. For example, in a study of postnatal care there is little point in collecting data about antenatal admissions, ultrasound scans or booking visits. The key is to identify which aspects of care *might* change and collect only relevant resource use information. If in any doubt, costs should be estimated, at least crudely, to allow later 'what if' analysis. This approach is called Sensitivity Analysis (see Box 7.5).

Once the question of which data will be collected has been addressed, resource use profiles can be built up for the two systems of care. Remember that data have to be collected on the existing model of service delivery to act as a baseline for comparison. Data collection is discussed later in the chapter. Resource use profiles can then be costed, using local costs. Cost information will come from a variety of sources, but is not always easy to understand. The most practical way of obtaining cost information is through the finance department of the Trust but these may not be provided in the

Box 7.5: Sensitivity analysis

In any evaluation, it is crucial to undertake sensitivity analysis on both the costs and benefits, particularly if assumptions have had to be made. Sensitivity analysis is a collection of techniques for exploring uncertainty in economic evaluations. Uncertainty can arise for many reasons: some inputs may have been excluded from the analysis because they are thought not to be affected, some costs or outcomes may have been based on data which may not be representative. Where evidence about costs and outcomes is collected in the local context, uncertainty may arise because data are sampled, and there is variation from case to case. Prices of inputs may vary, and where future costs or outcomes are included in the analysis, there is uncertainty about the best discount factor to use.

Sensitivity analysis is simply recalculation of the cost difference or cost effectiveness based on new assumptions about specific prices, input quantities or outcomes. This can take account of one or more aspects of uncertainty, and can become quite a complex modelling process where the analysis includes variation of many interdependent factors. This methodology is still the subject of research by health economists. A useful summary of sensitivity analysis in economic evaluation is given in an article by Briggs and his colleagues (1994).

An example of two-way sensitivity analysis in assessment of cost difference arising from policy of early versus delayed selective surfactant for babies at high risk of respiratory distress syndrome Based on the results of the OSIRIS trial (OSIRIS Collaborative Group, 1992) early use of surfactant is estimated to reduce neonatal deaths by 3.3 deaths in every 100 babies treated, when compared to delayed selective treatment. However there is uncertainty around this estimate – the 95 per cent confidence interval in the effect on mortality suggests this could be from no change to a reduction of 6.7 deaths per 100 babies treated. The expected change in cost of surfactant and neonatal care per baby is estimated to be an additional £314 per baby, however, based on uncertainty about doses, bed use and daily costs in the neonatal unit, this could be between £234 and £394. On the basis of the mid point estimates, the cost associated with each additional survivor is £9,515. But 'extreme scenario' sensitivity analysis shows that this estimate might be as low as £3,493, and it is also possible that, if deaths are not reduced that no benefit is gained and that costs are therefore increased for no purpose (Briggs, Sculpher and Buxton, 1994).

form needed for the specific question. Ward costs are usually disaggregated into elements such as midwifery, medical staff, pharmacy supplies, cleaning, laundry, and into fixed, semi-fixed and variable costs. Similar breakdowns will be available for out-patients, theatres and community midwifery. An example of a typical breakdown of costs into fixed, semi-fixed and variable is shown in Table 7.2. In this example, the majority of costs are hospital costs; these account for 61 per cent of the total service cost. However, if the pattern of care were to change to caseload midwifery, for example, as at Queen Charlotte's (Piercy et al., 1996) then the share of community as a proportion of the whole would be much higher. In addition, well over half of the service costs are classed as semi-fixed. This is explained by the high proportion of the total cost accounted for by midwifery salaries. Midwives, in costing terms, are counted as semi-fixed costs. For diagnostic tests, prices will often be quoted, but in the NHS, costs are supposed to equal prices, so in theory it will not make any difference.

	Whole service %	Hospital %	Community %	Out-patients %
Fixed	23	18	25	42
Semi-fixed	72	77	73	50
Variable	5	5	2	8
Proportion of total cost	100	61	22	17

Table 7.2: Fixed, semi-fixed and variable costs – a typical example

The interpretation of costs is not straightforward, nor which aspects of cost to use. Discussions with experienced evaluators are often likely to be of benefit in helping researchers understand the issues. For whole service evaluations it is probably better to call in the 'experts' or at least talk the process through before setting out.

When choosing an option for providing care, it is not just the average costs that matter, but the cost (and benefits) of providing more care when the service is already provided for some clients. This is known as marginal cost, and is not always the same as average costs. As long as there is spare capacity in staffing and space, marginal cost would include only the variable part of cost. In the longer run, marginal costs of additional clients may be nearer to average total costs, as sustained increase in workload usually needs more staff and space. The aim of economic evaluation of any type is not only to decide whether to provide a service at all, but to discover the level of service, or 'margin', where resources could achieve greater benefit in a different use. A related term often used in economic evaluation is marginal or *incremental* cost-effectiveness. This refers to the *additional* cost of achieving an *additional* unit of benefit when comparing one form of care with another (see Box 7.6).

Costs are local

Finally, researchers need to be aware that costs obtained locally will only have direct relevance in that context. Costs may not be directly transferable from hospital to hospital. The reasons for this are numerous, and include:

- Trusts can negotiate their own terms and conditions for staff;
- overheads will vary between Trusts;
- Trusts will have different structures and organizational policies, even within maternity departments;
- skill-mix will be different;
- wards will be different sizes;
- facilities will not be the same (buildings, layout, equipment);
- hospitals will have different workloads.

However, resource utilization may be easier to generalize. For example, if a model of care requires eight antenatal visits, the resource use associated with these eight visits may be the same in other units. In other words, they can duplicate the system of care and copy protocols. However, the unit *costs* of providing the care can be different, and Trusts will be able to apply local costs to any pattern of care. In reality though, a pattern of care may well employ somewhat different resources in different settings because of the small local variations in needs and infrastructure.

Benefits

Economic evaluation needs to consider what the benefits of the intervention or of the new method of service delivery will be as well as the costs.

How to choose the measure of effectiveness or benefit

The chosen measure of benefit will depend on what the objectives of the programme or treatment are. If the aim of the evaluation is merely to find out the least costly way of providing a service, such as the organization of midwife teams, taking the amount of care delivered (such as the number of antenatal visits per woman) to be constant, then benefit or effectiveness does not need to be considered. If the objective of the study is to estimate the benefit of the scheme in money terms (e.g. costs of treatments avoided), then cost-benefit analysis is appropriate. More likely, however, analysis of maternity issues will take into account non-financial objectives. These might include:

- meeting *Changing Childbirth* targets
- reducing the requirement for pain relief and other interventions in labour
- enhancing consumer satisfaction
- reducing the number of inductions necessary
- reducing the number of antenatal visits.

Some of these are outcomes; some are measure of process but all are objectives which can be measured. Although these are not financial outcomes, some evaluations attempt to value them in money terms by asking what society or individuals would pay to have or avoid the outcome; such studies are known as willingness-to-pay studies.

Benefits can also be measured in natural units, for example, an evaluation of Down's Syndrome screening might take as an outcome the number of cases detected. This is an example of an intermediate output. However, it must be shown that intermediate outputs have some value, and be translatable into health (and cost) effects. In Box 7.6 there is an example of an economic evaluation of screening for Down's Syndrome which also illustrates the principle of marginal cost.

Box 7.6: Marginal costs

One way of explaining the role of marginal costs in evaluation is to consider a programme of screening for Down's Syndrome. Marginal costs, in this context, represent the cost of identifying an extra case of Down's Syndrome through a biochemical pregnancy screening programme compared to screening using maternal age. In the example here (Torgerson, 1995) women over 35 were investigated further and the cost was £28,820 for each affected pregnancy detected. The biochemical screening programme covered women of all ages. For women aged over 35, the cost of additional detection is:

<u>cost of new programme *minus* cost of old programme</u>
new detections *minus* old detections

This gives us the *marginal* or *incremental* costs of detection.

For the remaining women, where there was no previous programme, the cost of detection is:

<u>cost of programme</u>
new detections

Torgerson analysed the marginal cost of detections by age band and found the following results:

Age band	Marginal cost (£)
35 and over	3,854*
30–34	34,381
25–29	47,885
20–24	89,831
less than 20	174,449

*compared to maternal age screening alone for over 35s.

The falling cost as age increases is due to the increasing risk of Down's Syndrome for babies of older mothers.

It is worth noting that effects other than the foreseen effects may be obtained. Researchers should not ignore these effects. For example, in a study looking at the impact on midwifery workload, an intervention which alters the way in which midwives work may also produce benefits such as increased patient satisfaction. If the new scheme proved more expensive, then the increased cost can be measured against the additional benefits, and a management decision taken concerning whether the benefits are worth the costs. The better the evidence about the benefits, on the one hand, and the non-financial 'costs' of a new scheme (things such as poorer health outcomes or unhappiness), on the other hand, the better the economic evaluation. The issues discussed earlier in the book about the quality of evidence produced by different methods are also important here (see Chapters 3 and 4 in particular).

As we have described, economic evaluation compares costs and outcomes in different ways. Where a form of care affects several different outcomes in different ways, or if two aspects of care with very different outcomes are compared, then some way is needed to sum up the overall change in 'benefit' in order to compare the change in benefit with changes in costs. Two examples might illustrate this. First, two methods for repairing perineal trauma after childbirth using different suture materials which are equally acceptable in terms of post-partum pain can both reduce the (frequent) need for short term stitch removal and increase the (less frequent) need for resuturing. How should midwives choose which is preferable? Some method is needed to weigh up the conflicting outcomes. Secondly, a health authority might want to compare a maternity programme with a programme for care of sick elderly people. Again, some way is needed to help decision makers to weigh up the possible gains in babies' and women's health and women's satisfaction with the health gain of the older population.

Methods proposed by health economists all attempt to find the value which people apply to different health outcomes and therefore to different services. This includes direct monetary valuation – asking people what they think is the right amount to pay for a particular service (the willingness to pay approach), and methods not requiring money values which ask people to give relative valuations of different health states (utility measurement) and which are used in estimation of so-called 'quality adjusted life years' or QALYs. Although the principle of economic benefit measurement is clearly important, the methods for such estimation are subject to debate and are at varying stages of development as research tools. If readers plan to try to estimate economic benefits in either of these ways, they would be well advised to seek the help of a health economist with experience in this aspect of evaluation.

How to collect data about benefits

Many of the outcome measures such as patient satisfaction, impact on service providers, clinical standards, safety and efficacy are discussed elsewhere in this book, along with methods of data collection. It is not proposed to discuss these in this section. Hospital information systems contain some outcome and plenty of process information. It might be possible, for example, to obtain information relating to method of delivery, use of pain relief, APGAR scores, and the requirement for neonatal care from hospital data sets. Other information, such as rates of breastfeeding and incidence of postnatal depression, will require a specific study to be designed to collect the data.

Resource use information

This section considers three important issues, namely:

- what information do you need?
- what sources are available?
- how might data be analysed?

Data sources which will be considered include hospital data sets, casenote data and developing data collection tools to fill in any gaps which may be apparent.

Which data about resources are needed in evaluation?

Clearly the level and detail of data collection will depend on the issue which is being addressed. For example, for a study evaluating short postnatal length of stay, data would be required concerning postnatal length of stay, community postnatal care (since care is being shifted from hospital to community) and outcome information such as readmission rates and complications for mother and baby. Psychological well-being may also be considered important. On the other hand, a study considering changes in the organization of midwifery care, to increase continuity of care, would need to consider the impact on midwifery workload, hence changes to the number and grade of midwives involved, together with a data collection tool to measure continuity of care, perhaps noting the number of different people a woman sees during her pregnancy.

A general rule is only to collect data which are of direct relevance. An important task therefore is to identify what the impact of the change might be and where resource use patterns are likely be changed; for example, hospital to community, number of diagnostic tests. You also need to decide which outcomes are appropriate. In all cases, data should not be collected on resources or outcomes which are not affected. For example, in an evaluation of postnatal community care, data relating to antenatal and hospital intrapartum care are not needed. Collecting them will at best mean that the study will take longer, and will almost certainly lead to unnecessary complications.

Information sources

The sources considered in this section relate to resource use and basic outcome information. Data relating to women's experience of care are covered elsewhere in the book. The aim of this section is to provide an overview for each data source covering:

- information that can be obtained;
- method and ease of obtaining the data;
- method of analysis;
- advantages and problems of this method of data collection.

HOSPITAL MINIMUM DATASETS (MAINLY IN-PATIENT DATA)

a)   Information available

All hospitals are required to collect basic information relating to the work they undertake – the hospital activity. This information is a useful starting point when considering data requirements since it is readily available. Generally, hospital minimum datasets relate to in-patient activity and will include information for each admission relating to:

- reason for admission (diagnosis) and admission method;
- procedures undertaken (including method of delivery);
- length of stay;
- postcode of residence;
- admitting consultant and patient's GP;
- discharge information.

It is often possible, given that each woman has a unique hospital number, to obtain complete records of in-patient care for any patient, and to link this to other available information and to casenote analysis. These data will tell a researcher how often a woman has been admitted to hospital, the reason why she was admitted, how long she stayed and what happened whilst she was there. Many hospitals also use specially designed information systems for maternity care (discussed in more detail in the chapter on information systems) which can also provide useful indicators of resource use.

b)   Obtaining the data

These data are held centrally on a database controlled by the hospital information department. For research purposes, it is usually necessary to request the data from the director of information or a senior information officer, even for staff who work in the Trust. Typically, information will be provided on computer disk to allow for analysis to take place. Normally, there are few difficulties in getting access to this information, though due to pressure of workload on information technology (IT) departments, it may take some time.

It is often necessary to specify how the information is to be supplied, but the IT department will be able to advise on the appropriate format, depending on the proposed method of analysis and available computer facilities. If detailed data analysis is not required, then the IT department will often be able to present basic information such as average length of stay or method of delivery in summary form. This is easier than the researcher undertaking their own analysis, though it is likely to take longer for the summary statistics to be produced. Again, the IT department will be able to advise but they will only be able to do this with a full understanding of the aims of the study.

c)   Analysis

If the researcher obtains a database, the method of analysis is likely to involve a computer. Ideally, a statistical package such as SPSS would be used, but a spreadsheet system will do as long as it is fairly modern, can read the data (check with the information department) and can produce basic statistics such as means and frequencies. If any doubt persists with regard to what to do or how to do it, then contacting management information within the Trust is a good starting point.

Information worth obtaining from a minimum dataset includes:

- number of antenatal and intrapartum admissions;
- mean and median length of stay of antenatal admissions and intrapartum admissions;
- method of delivery (percentage of all deliveries);
- nature and frequency of complications;
- mean and median postnatal length of stay;
- out-patient activity.

In all cases, either request antenatal and intrapartum episodes in separate files or be prepared to split them up yourself: antenatal admissions are those with no 'method of delivery' OPCS-4 code. The two *cannot* be analysed together (for obvious reasons). Information with respect to procedures and diagnoses is often in code form: ICD-9 or ICD-10 codes for diagnoses (International Classification of Diseases), OPCS-4 for procedures. These will need to be 'decoded'. The hospital information department or the maternity business manager/clinical director is likely to have the ICD code book and the OPCS manual. Some Trusts are moving to Healthcare Resource Groups (HRG) as a measure of activity as an alternative to procedure codes. These are simpler and are classified by method of delivery, but are not yet well developed for antenatal events and admissions.

d)   Points to note

Hospital information systems are only as good as the quality of the data entered. If data entry is poor or unreliable, then the information received will be of doubtful value. Given that the minimum dataset is supposed to be used for calculating and planning future workload and for contract monitoring, it ought to be reasonably accurate – often though it is not. It is certainly worth checking for accuracy. One method is to compare the number of deliveries recorded on the information dataset with the records kept in delivery suite. The two should be identical (or at least close). Method of delivery can also be compared.

It is also possible that out-patient data may be available, though these are more likely to be of doubtful quality, and the researcher must make sure he/she knows what an out-patient dataset contains. Out-patient datasets can include some or all of consultant out-patient attendances and parentcraft classes. Equally, antenatal admissions may include day cases, attendances at an antenatal day assessment unit, visits to a fetal monitoring unit and so forth. It is prudent to check with the information department what is included and how to tell what is being measured. An example of the potential pitfalls associated with hospital data is outlined in Box 7.7.

Box 7.7: Information definitions

It is always prudent to check with information departments about what is included under each data item, and what exactly is being measured. This is particularly important when the information system is relatively new. For example, in the Queen Charlotte's evaluation (Piercy et al., 1996), at first sight the data indicated a high number of admissions which were counted as day cases. Indeed, around half the women were 'credited' with a day case admission. However, we were aware that day case admissions were rare. On consultation with the information department, it was found that appointments at the fetal monitoring unit had been coded as day cases. This anomaly had been removed by the time that data for the final report had been received and analysed.

Finally, analysing hospital information alone is rarely enough for economic evaluation. Many gaps will be left to fill from other data sources, such as casenotes. Specific 'data capture' tools may also have to be developed.

CASENOTE ANALYSIS

a)   Information available

Hospital datasets contain broad information about hospital activity, and occasionally more specific information relating to out-patient attendances, diagnostic tests and investigations. However, a potentially more reliable source of such information is patient/hospital casenotes. Indeed, hospital casenotes can provide a wealth of information including:

- test and investigations;
- ultrasound scans;
- out-patient attendances;
- drugs prescribed in hospital;
- pain relief during delivery;
- induction;
- reason for assisted delivery/caesarean section;
- records of antenatal and postnatal care.

In addition basic outcome measures such as Apgar scores, postnatal complications and rates of breastfeeding may be available.

b)   Obtaining the data

Casenotes are usually straightforward to obtain, as long as researchers do not wish to go back too far in time. Permission from research ethics committees may need to be obtained. It may take some time and negotiation to gain access to records, partly because records staff may be very busy and may not be able to give priority to research studies. A data capture form will be required so all the information can be retrieved from a set of casenotes at one time. Hence, before the researcher starts investigating casenotes, they should know what information they are seeking. Otherwise, unnecessary work and duplication of effort may result, and casenote analysis is not the most interesting of tasks at the best of times. Furthermore, a well-designed data capture form will make analysis much easier. Bias can arise from missing casenotes: these often relate to cases where the notes are being held for an investigation, or where something went wrong.

c)   Analysis

If a lot of information is needed or if there are large numbers of casenotes involved, the best method of undertaking analysis is to enter the data on to a computer, either on to a spreadsheet or through creating a database. Creation of databases is probably the best way but will require some computing expertise: if the dataset is not too large then entering data on a spreadsheet will probably work equally well, certainly for basic analysis. Furthermore it is possible to read data from spreadsheets such as Quattro Pro into statistical packages, so more complex analysis can be undertaken. However, this can be a difficult exercise, so ask for advice from IT or computer service departments if appropriate. Alternatively, research organizations specializing in clinical audit or economic evaluation might be able to assist, and would also be able to offer advice about:

- the best way of undertaking the analysis;
- what questions to ask;
- what statistical tests are relevant;
- how to undertake them.

However, if the evaluation is small and focuses on only one or two aspects of care, it may not be necessary to use computers, particularly if resources used are simply being noted and counted, e.g. number of ultrasound scans.

d)   Points to note

Casenote analysis is likely to be time-consuming for a number of reasons. It takes some time to identify and find the relevant casenotes, and then a lot of time to get the data out. There is no standard format for the presentation and structure of casenotes; some hospital notes will be easier to analyse than others. There are sources of bias in analysis of casenotes. For example, 'interesting' or complicated cases may be missing. However, it is likely that much of the data required will be contained in the casenotes, particularly in relation to actions carried out in a hospital setting such as tests, out-patient attendances and intrapartum care. Casenotes are less useful for analysis of care taking place outside hospital, for example home antenatal visits. Information is likely to be incomplete and not all actions will be recorded. Furthermore, hospital casenotes will not contain any information relating to primary care. To investigate this, GP notes may be required.

e)   GP casenotes

GP casenotes will contain information relating to the care women receive in the primary care environment. If you are planning to use GP casenotes then you need to bear in mind the following:

*   consent has to be obtained from each GP;
*   in any one year, each GP is likely to deal with only 20 to 30 maternity cases;
*   casenotes may not record contacts with members of the primary health care team other than the GP;
*   it is difficult to link GP and hospital records;
*   maternity information will be mixed with other information so identifying maternity contacts may be hard.

If it is necessary to use these notes, then analysis is the same as for hospital casenotes. Some GP practices now have computerized information systems, and these may well make it easier to look at care in both the hospital and community setting.

Other new data collection

Often, it is likely that information required may not be held in either hospital datasets or casenotes. Examples of such information includes assessment of midwife workload, duration of contacts and number of people involved in the delivery of care. In such cases, it will be necessary for the researcher to collect the data using their own data collection tool. Clearly, data can be collected on virtually any topic which is observable and measurable. To obtain the data, three key questions must be addressed. Firstly, the researcher must decide precisely which data are required. If the researcher is unsure, then a pilot study is a method of finding out whether the data collected are useful, and whether anything has been missed. As with casenote analysis, do not collect data you do not plan to use.

Secondly, the method of data collection must be established. There is a range of alternatives, including direct observation, diaries for mothers having care, increasing existing routine data collection, and structured surveys of managers responsible for key resources. In all cases, data collection forms need to be designed. This must be done with a view to analysis; simple forms from which it is easy to extract data are always best.

Thirdly, it needs to be established who will collect the data. This may not always be the researcher. If data are collected by somebody else, then the form must be short, easy to understand and to complete and must not place too great a burden on the person(s) collecting the data. Forms which take more than a minute to fill in after each observation (e.g. antenatal care contacts) are too long! This method of obtaining data often places burdens on staff (or patients) who are outside the research team. In all such cases, it is vital to explain the purpose of the study, making it clear why this particular information is important, and keeping people informed of progress of the study and results. If the researcher is to collect the data, then the whole process is likely to be time consuming and this must be taken into account when assessing likely project timescales and costs. However, this method is often the best way of obtaining community based data and to inform issues such as continuity of care and carer.

Summary of sources for data on resource use

Box 7.8 gives an example of combining data from several different sources when looking at costs and Table 7.3 summarizes the points covered in this section.

Box 7.8: Gathering multicentre cost data to estimate costs of alternative policies for surfactant use in neonatal care

It has now been shown that surfactant reduces the risk of death and chronic lung disease in pre-term babies at high risk of respiratory distress (RDS). It is, however, an expensive product, at over £400 per baby treated. Two multicentre trials comparing policies of giving surfactant at different times and doses have incorporated measures of the use of neonatal hospital care, in terms of doses of surfactant and days at different levels of intensity of care. A group of paediatricians and economists involved in these trials have surveyed the costs of care in UK neonatal units taking part in the trials. This involved gathering data from routine sources about the number of days of intensive, special and nursery care provided in each unit, and using a questionnaire to the senior nurses and business managers about the units' resources and costs. The cost of care at each level was then estimated using a statistical modelling method to estimate a generally applicable relationship between total cost in each unit and the number of days, and the proportion at each level of care. The unit costs derived in this way provide a basis for comparing the costs of resource differences arising from different surfactant policies. Early, prophylactic, surfactant use, when compared to delayed selective surfactant for babies who have developed RDS, reduces the requirement for intensive (ventilator) care by one day, although overall length of stay is not different. The evidence so far available from the cost models suggests that this may offset the increased cost of surfactant resulting from the policy (Mugford, 1995).

	Hospital minimum data set	Other hospital data (e.g. pathology, delivery suite)*	Casenotes	Original data collection

Information attainable	1. Inpatient activity
	  – procedures
	  – diagnosis
	  – length of stay.
		1. Diagnostic testing
		  – pathology
		  – ultrasound
		2. Delivery suite information
		  – pain relief
		  – complications
		  – method of delivery.
			1. All diagnostic information
			2. All delivery suite information
			3. Times of transfers between wards
			4. Background information on women: parity, ethnicity, maternal history
			5. Outpatient contacts, community ante/postnatal contacts
			6. Outcome data.
				1. Anything, but particularly useful for recording
				  – 'community' based care, e.g. home visits
				  – number of staff present at contacts
				  – continuity of care information.

Method of obtaining data	Data held by the hospital information department.	Data held by relevant local managers.	Notes held by medical records, GPs or consultants.	Individual data capture sheets. Depends on amount of information required.
Ease of obtaining data	Straightforward in theory if staff are co-operative.	Straightforward in theory if staff are co-operative.	Finding notes is not always easy. A data capture form is required.	Requires co-operation of staff who will collect the data.
Method of analysis	Computer analysis – spreadsheets – statistical packages.	Computer analysis – spreadsheets – statistical packages.	Entry onto database and computer analysis is the best way to handle lots of data.	Entry onto database and computer analysis is the best way to handle lots of data.
Advantages	Minimum data sets are comparable across hospitals and over time (usually).	Avoids casenote analysis if available.	Detailed information, best source of outcome data.	Can collect whatever information is wanted subject to time, co-operation of staff and money for research.
Potential problems	Information can be of doubtful quality as it depends on accurate data entry. Limited range of information Management not research information.	Information can be of doubtful quality as it depends on accurate data entry. Systems different in different providers. Management not research information.	Time consuming. May need ethical approval. Notes may need to be interpreted. Can be complicated to analyse.	Very time consuming. Requires co-operation from many staff if not collected by researcher. Complicated to analyse.

Table 7.3: Information sources for resource use

* 'Other hospital data' relates to databases which may be already in existence. These will vary from hospital to hospital. The examples here relating to pathology and delivery suite are illustrative. If such information is not present, casenote analysis will be required.

Finding unit cost data

So far the sources we have described have been for information mainly about quantities of resource use as a result of different policies. The final step of data collection in cost comparisons is to place a value on each item of resource use. This information may come from a variety of sources. The following examples illustrate this.

- Staff costs: if resource use has been estimated in terms of hours of staff input required for a particular service, then the staff cost per hour can be estimated as the hourly employment cost measured by salary plus additional employer's costs. The additional costs are the costs to the employer of providing employment benefits such as pensions, sickness payments, training and so on. The finance officer of a Trust will know what the average cost is for any staff group.

- Materials and disposables: these can be difficult to cost, but increasingly, supplies departments have costed lists of items, and it is becoming more common for costs to be specified on requisition sheets. Be careful in interpreting costs of items that are used more than once: the aim is to assess the cost of the use of the item per single use.

- Laboratory and diagnostic tests: if you are lucky, your Trust will have a costing and pricing section where costs of items from different 'service' departments have been estimated in detail. It is seldom worth setting up a detailed study of lab costs for the purpose of maternity costing, and so rules of thumb are often used, based on average costs of similar types of test. Laboratory and other departmental managers are usually a helpful source in this investigation.

- Drug costs: hospital pharmacies are usually very well informed about the costs of the drugs they supply. Prices for all prescription drugs are listed in the Drug Tariff which will be readily available from hospital pharmacies and is updated every month. Information about drug costs is also published in the British National Formulary, which is updated regularly and supplied to all prescribers. This gives a cost range for each drug which is probably sufficiently precise for most costing studies.

- 'Hotel costs' and overheads of being in hospital: the average daily cost of non-clinical services can be derived very crudely from the total cost of these services divided by the number of patient days in the hospital. This does not reflect different demands on non-clinical services by different patients or wards (such as laundry use, or heating requirements), and in particular cases (such as neonatal intensive care wards) more detailed costing may need to be done. Discussion with the unit accountant may help to clarify if the departments you are costing are likely to be atypical.

Writing up the study

Once the data have been collected, they need to be analysed, then drawn together. The decision rules for undertaking evaluation were outlined earlier, and are summarized here:

Cost Benefit Analysis: Accept A if the benefits of A exceed the costs of A

Cost Effectiveness Analysis: Accept A if the relative benefits of B to A are not worth the additional costs of B relative to A.

If under cost-effectiveness analysis, one of the options is both less expensive and confers more benefits, the decision is clear. More commonly, with CEA, one option will be more beneficial but also more expensive. This is where a management decision is required, and all the researcher can and should do is to present the evidence. Remember, economic evaluation is only an *aid* to decision making! Interpretation of the results is a management decision, though researchers can (and do) influence this decision in the way the study is presented.

Summary

This section outlines the key steps required to undertake an economic evaluation.

a) *Decide on the aims and objectives*
- set any hypotheses;
- pose the relevant economic questions;
- identify key audience.

b) *Identify the appropriate form of analysis*
- cost-benefit analysis or cost-effectiveness analysis;
- decide how to measure the benefits of the intervention.

c) *Data collection*
- identify which data need to be collected (with reference to the question addressed);
- identify any data sources and any gaps;
- decide a method of data analysis;
- design any data capture tools and databases (get a computer expert to help here);
- locate case notes (and obtain ethical approval if needed);
- collect the data.

d) *Analyse the data*
- develop resource use profiles;
- cost resource use profiles;
- identify and quantify the benefits/outcomes;
- undertake the cost benefit/cost effectiveness according to the decision rules set out here;
- undertake sensitivity analysis.

e) *Present the study*
- identify the audience: managers, clinicians, professional journals;
- write the report and prepare an executive summary.

At all stages and particularly in the design phase, inexperienced and occasional researchers should not be afraid to ask for advice either internally to understand what is happening (clinicians, managers, finance staff), or externally for advice (academic units, other researchers). Even experienced researchers need to ask for help sometimes!

Box 7.9: Sources of help and advice in health economics in the UK

The UK **Health Economists Study Group** (HESG) is a forum and network for health economists, administered from the Health Economics Research Unit, University Medical Buildings, Foresterhill, Aberdeen AB9 2ZD, to whom all enquiries should be directed. This group compiles an annual list of research interests of members.

National Health Service Health Economics Group. This group aims to facilitate and promote the use of Health Economics in the NHS by dissemination and brokerage of information about health economics activities in the NHS, both in progress and at a conceptual stage, by newsletter, local and national meetings. All NHS employees are eligible to join and persons from other relevant organizations (such as local authorities or the Civil Service) can be considered for associate membership. The group welcomes any individual from these sectors who is interested in promoting health economics. The Chair is Dr M Jennings, Senior Lecturer and Honorary Consultant Physician in Health Care for Elderly People, Northern General Hospital NHS Trust, Herries Road, Sheffield S5 7AU, to whom all enquiries should be directed. There are also regional and national groups in different areas of the UK including Scotland, Northern Ireland, London and the Anglia and Oxford Region.

References

Briggs, A., Sculpher, M., Buxton, M. (1994). 'Uncertainty in the economic evaluation of health care technologies: the role of sensitivity analysis'. *Health Economics*, Vol. 3, pp. 95–104.

Health Services Management Centre and Birmingham Women's Health Care Trust (1996). *Woman-Focused Care – At What Cost? A Resource Manual.* Enquiries to: Midwifery Administration, Birminham Women's Health Care NHS Trust, Birmingham B15 2TG.

Mugford, M. (1995). 'Cost-effectivenss of policies for surfactant use based on the results of the OSIRIS trial: a preliminary analysis'. *Neonatal Monitor,* Vol. 12, pp. 10–12.

Mugford, M. (1996). *How Does the Method of Cost Estimation Affect the Assessment of Cost-effectiveness in Health Care?* DPhil Thesis. Oxford University.

OSIRIS Collaborative Group (1992). 'Early versus delayed neonatal administration of a synthetic surfactant – the judgement of OSIRIS'. *Lancet,* Vol. 340, pp. 1363–69.

Piercy, J., Wilson, D., Chapman, P. (1996). *Evaluation of One-to One Midwifery Practice.* York: York Health Economics Consortium, York University.

Ratcliffe, J., Ryan, M., Tucker, J. (1996). 'The costs of alternative types of routine antenatal care for low risk women: shared care vs care by general practitioners and community midwives'. *Journal of Health Services Research and Policy,* Vol. 1, pp. 135–140.

Ryan, M., Ratcliffe, J., Tucker, J. (1997). 'Using willingness to pay to value alternative models of antenatal care'. *Social Science and Medicine,* Vol. 44, pp. 371–80.

Sculpher, M., Drummond, M., Buxton, M.J. (1997). 'Economic evaluation in health care research and development'. *Journal of Health Services Research and Policy,* Vol. 2, pp. 26–30.

Torgerson, D.J. (1996). 'Cost effectiveness of Down's syndrome screening'. In: Gradsinskas, J.D., Ward, R.H. (Eds). *Screening for Down's Syndrome in the First Trimester. Thirty Second Study Group RCOG.* London: RCOG Publications.

Tucker, J.S., Hall, M.H., Howie, P.W., Reid, M.E., Barbour, R.S., Florey, C. du V. et al. (1996). 'Should obstetricians see women with normal pregnancies? A multicentre randomized controlled trial of routine antenatal care by general practitioners and midwives compared to obstetrician led care'. *British Medical Journal,* Vol. 312, pp. 554–59.

Further reading

Bell, J. (1993). *Doing Your Research Project. A Guide for First-Time Researchers in Education and Social Sciences.* Buckingham: Open University Press.

Drummond, M.F., Stoddart, G.L., Torrance, G.W. (1987). *Methods for Economic Evaluation in Health Care.* Oxford: Oxford University Press.

Howard, S., McKell, D., Mugford, M., Grant, A. (1995). 'Cost-effectiveness of different approaches to perineal suturing'. *British Journal of Midwifery,* Vol. 3, pp. 587–605.

Hundley, V., Cruickshank, F., Lang, G., Glazener, C., Milne, J., Turner, M. et al. (1994). 'Midwife managed delivery unit: a randomized controlled comparison with consultant led care'. *British Medical Journal,* Vol. 309, pp. 1400–1404.

Hundley, V., Donaldson, C. (1995). 'Costs of intrapartum care in a midwife managed delivery unit and a consultant supervised labour'. *Midwifery,* 11, pp. 103–109.

Jefferson, T., Demicheli, V., Mugford, M. (1996). *Elementary Economic Evaluation in Health Care.* London: British Medical Journal Publishing Group.

Mugford, M., Drummond, M.F. (1989). 'The role of economics in the evaluation of care'. In: Chalmers, I., Enkin, M., Keirse, M.J. (Eds). *Effective Care in Pregnancy and Childbirth.* 1st edition. Oxford: Oxford University Press.

Mugford, M., Kingston, J., Chalmers, I. (1989). 'Reducing the incidence of infection after caesarian section: implications of prophylaxis with antibotics for hospital resources'. *British Medical Journal,* Vol. 299, pp. 1003–1006.

Mugford, M. (1993). *Steroids for Women Expected to Deliver Prematurely. Estimates of Impact of Wider Use.* Oxford: Oxford Regional Health Authority.

Mugford, M., Piercy, J., Chalmers, I. (1991). 'Cost implications of different approaches to the prevention of respiratory distress syndrome'. *Archives of Disease in Childhood,* Vol. 66, pp. 757–764.

Mugford, M., Mlika-Cabanne, N., Bréart, G. (1992). 'EC trial of management of labour in primiparous women: first report from the economic evaluation'. In: Kaminski, M. (Ed). *Evaluation in Pre-, Peri- and Post-Natal Care Delivery Systems: A European Concerted Action.* Paris: Inserm.

Twaddle, S., Harper, V. (1992). 'An economic evaluation of daycare in the management of hypertension in pregnancy'. *British Journal of Obstetrics and Gynaecology,* Vol. 99, pp. 459–463.

CHAPTER EIGHT

Information Systems

Mary Ness, Pam Dobson, Alison Macfarlane, Jo Garcia, Rona Campbell

The aim of this chapter is to provide a guide to the kinds of information systems that are available, both at national and local level, and to explore how these can best be harnessed to support evaluations. To illustrate how routine information systems can be used effectively in an evaluation we begin by describing, in Box 8.1, how a computerized maternity information system supplied much of the data required for an evaluation of a pilot midwifery led care scheme. While most of the people using this book will probably be concerned with evaluations at a unit or district level, there is still a need to set local findings in context by comparing them, where possible, with national data. The chapter therefore includes a brief guide to national information systems. This is followed by a review of the different types of local computer systems which might be relevant in an evaluation of maternity services. It also discusses how to find out what systems are available and appraise whether they can provide the data required. In units which do not have a suitable maternity information system, the search for one can be prompted by the desire to undertake an evaluation. Likewise, the failure of an existing system to provide data for an evaluation may also increase pressure to invest in a new system. For this reason the final part of this chapter gives some advice on what to look for in maternity information systems.

The experience described in Box 8.1 relates to one particular Trust but there are undoubtedly others in which similar things have happened. This example illustrates how, before starting to collect information for use in evaluations, it is essential to check if the information is already available through routine systems within the service. Since care givers and other staff already spend a great deal of time recording information in individual records, in books like theatre or labour ward records and in computer systems, managers and researchers should only be asking staff to fill in extra forms for an evaluation if it is absolutely necessary. There are two advantages to using existing data. Firstly, doing this avoids duplication of effort, and secondly, using the data may improve their quality because staff who collect data will get feedback on their work.

Box 8.1: Using a maternity information system to evaluate a pilot midwife led care scheme

---

A pilot scheme to provide midwife led care throughout pregnancy and childbirth, for women thought to be at low risk of complications, was introduced in a combined hospital and community Trust. In order to evaluate the pilot scheme midwives began to collect data manually on birth outcomes and on the care given during labour and delivery. When the midwifery information systems co-ordinator became aware of this, it was pointed out that most of the information required was on the computerized maternity information system (MIS). All that was required was the addition of a new item to the system which identified whether women had been allocated to midwife led care, consultant led care or a control group. The evaluation was thus undertaken using data from the MIS.

As it was difficult to do detailed statistical analyses within the MIS, special files of data were downloaded from the system to a personal computer. The data analysis for the evaluation was then performed using the statistical package SPSS. Some of the data items required for the evaluation, such as the length of time spent on the labour ward, were not routinely entered on the MIS and therefore still had to be collected manually. Had there been earlier contact between those managing the MIS and those conducting the evaluation it should have been possible to adjust the system so that it included this information (Thomas, Personal communication).

National information systems

The registration of births and deaths by parents or next of kin is a major source of data on the subject. In England and Wales, birth and death statistics are compiled by the Office for National Statistics (ONS). This organization was formed on April 1 1996 when the Office of Population Censuses and Surveys (OPCS) merged with the Central Statistical Office. The ONS publishes brief summaries of national birth and infant mortality statistics, together with rates by region and district of residence, as soon as they become available. The ONS, like its predecessor the OPCS, publishes these statistics in a colour coded series of papers referred to as *Monitors*. Details of births are published in the series labelled FM1, which is colour coded yellow, and details of deaths in the DH3 series, colour coded dark blue. More detailed birth and infant mortality data are published at a later stage in 'annual reference volumes' which use the same series labelling and colour coding. Scotland and Northern Ireland have their own General Register Offices and their statistics are published in the Annual Report of the Registrar General for Scotland and the Annual Report of the Registrar General for Northern Ireland. These volumes of statistics are often available in specialized health or academic libraries. The government offices responsible for compiling and publishing relevant national data are listed in Box 8.2. For other points of contact in central government, see *Government Statistics: A Brief Guide to Sources*, a free publication available from the ONS Library in Newport.

Box 8.2: Sources of national data

National Health Service statistics
England: Department of Health
Skipton House, 80 London Road, London SE1 6LW.
Maternity statistics: 0171 972 5697
Workforce, finance and performance analysis statistics:
Quarry House, Quarry Hill, Leeds LS2 7UE
NHS medical staff statistics: 0113 254 5892
NHS non-medical staff statistics: 0113 254 5744
Finance statistics: 0113 254 5390

Wales: Welsh Office
Statistical Directorate, Crown Buildings, Cathays Park, Cardiff CF1 3NQ
Health statistics: 01222 825080

Scotland: Information and Statistics Division
Trinity Park House, South Trinity Road, Edinburgh EH5 3SQ
Customer liaison: 0131 551 8899   0131 551 8974

Northern Ireland: Department of Health and Social Services
Annexe 2, Castle Buildings, Stormont, Belfast BT4 3UD
Health service statistics in general: 01232 522800
Maternity statistics from child health systems: 01232 522591

Birth and death registration statistics:
England and Wales: Office for National Statistics
1 Drummond Gate, London SW1 2QQ
Infant and perinatal mortality: 0171 533 5207
Fertility statistics: 0171 533 5113/5117
Surveys Including Infant Feeding Survey: 0171 533 5316
NHS Survey Advice Centre: 0171 533 5331

Segensworth Road, Titchfield, Fareham, Hampshire PO15 5RR.
Population estimates: 01329 813318   01329 813281
Census enquiries: 01329 813800

Scotland: General Register Office
New Register House, West Register Street, Edinburgh EH12 7TF
Population, vital events and census enquiries: 0131 314 4266

Northern Ireland: Northern Ireland Statistics and Research Agency
General Register Office, Oxford House, 49–55 Chichester St, Belfast BT1 4HL
Population and vital statistics: 01232 252032
Census Office, Arches Centre, 11–13 Bloomfield Avenue, Belfast BT5 5HD
General enquiries: 01232 526087

'Government statistics, a brief guide to sources':
Copies can be obtained from: The Library, Office for National Statistics,
Cardiff Road, Newport NP9 1XG.   01633 812973   Fax: 01633 81259

At an early stage in the annual publications process, the ONS compiles more detailed summaries of local birth and death rates and sends health authorities and local authorities these summaries for the populations of the geographical areas for which they are responsible. It also sells the complete sets of these tabulations for all districts in England and Wales on computer disks. Two sets of these tabulations are of particular relevance to people in the maternity services. Births in geographical areas are tabulated by mothers' ages, whether from inside or outside marriage, birthweight and place of birth, on the DVS2H tabulations. This information could be used, for example, in a local audit of births taking place at home, to check whether the number of such births identified in the audit was the same as the number registered by women living in the district.

Numbers and rates of live and stillbirths and infant mortality to women usually resident in each geographical area can be found on the DVS5H tabulations. These tabulations can be used by co-ordinators in the Confidential Enquiry into Stillbirths and Deaths in Infancy (CESDI) to see whether all the deaths which have been registered by parents are reported to the Enquiry.

Public health departments of health authorities in England and Wales are a good first point of contact when looking for these data locally. Similar data are likely to be available from health boards in Scotland and health and social services boards in Northern Ireland.

The ONS and the General Register Offices for Scotland and Northern Ireland are also responsible for collecting and publishing census data. The ONS also publishes data on abortions under the 1967 Act, congenital malformations, cancer registrations and communicable diseases. In Scotland these data are compiled by the Information and Statistics Division (ISD) of the National Health Service in Scotland. Apart from abortion statistics, some of these same data are published by the Department of Health and Social Services (DHSS) in Northern Ireland. NHS data for Wales are published by the Welsh Office.

The ONS also does large scale surveys on a number of topics. Some of these relate to health in general. For example, the General Household Survey, which has been done every year from 1971 to 1986, includes questions about health and about households with young children. In alternate years it asks about birth control. At the present time, the future of this useful survey is uncertain. A few ONS surveys are directly relevant to maternity care, notably its five yearly survey of infant feeding. The General Household Survey and the infant feeding surveys cover England, Wales and Scotland. Northern Ireland has a separate Continuous Household Survey and has more recently undertaken an infant feeding survey.

Statistics about finances, staffing and activities of the NHS are compiled and published annually by the health ministry of each country of the United Kingdom. Thus, the Department of Health produces *Health and Personal Social Services Statistics for England*, while the Welsh Office publishes *Health Statistics Wales*, the ISD publishes *Scottish Health Statistics* and the DHSS produces *Health and Personal Social Services Statistics for Northern Ireland*. ISD has brought Scottish maternity data from several sources together in a new publication *Births in Scotland* (1976–95).

Data from national information systems, which are mainly available on paper in an aggregated form, have a number of uses in local evaluations. They are often used as a source of national or regional figures which can be compared with local figures. In addition, some of them are used to produce local figures which can either complement data collected locally, or be used as a cross-check. In particular, some of the systems focus on data about the population of geographical areas and can be used to assess the extent to which the people who use a given maternity unit may be typical.

When auditing local trends, in induction rates or operative delivery rates for example, it is useful to set these against national trends. *Scottish Health Statistics* mentioned earlier includes data about these and other aspects of maternity care from the SMR2 maternity discharge system. Unfortunately, similar data cannot be found in the corresponding publications for England, Wales and Northern Ireland because of their poor quality and incompleteness (Macfarlane et al., 1995; Middle and Macfarlane, 1995a, b), although some data appear in reports of the House of Commons Health Committee. The Department of Health has now published a statistical bulletin containing data, which tries to make the best use of the data which have been collected through the Maternity Hospital Episode System (Department of Health, 1997).

The data available in the early 1980s were described in detail in Volume 1 of *Birth Counts: Statistics of Pregnancy and Childbirth* (Macfarlane and Mugford, 1984) while a second volume contained tables of data. A third volume is now being compiled to update these. Meanwhile, more up to date information can be found in a number of other shorter but more recent publications (Barron and Macfarlane, 1990; Thunhurst and Macfarlane, 1992; Macfarlane, 1994 a, b; Macfarlane et al., 1995). For a general guide to the full range of official statistics see the ONS *Guide to Official Statistics* (ONS, 1996).

Local information systems

There are a variety of local information systems which might contain information which could be used in an evaluation. Although the precise systems used vary considerably from one manufacturer to another, there are several broad categories of systems. These are described in Box 8.3.

Information systems are needed for a number of different purposes in maternity care. They can be used to monitor the clinical care given to an individual woman, by bringing together information about the visits made to various clinics and hospitals, the results of tests and procedures and the types of care given. Another use is to help in the planning of care. For example, it is possible to use the system to highlight potential risk factors when data are entered at the booking visit. Maternity information systems can also be used to generate a summary of the care and outcomes. One such summary is the notification of birth to the district health authority. This may be in paper or electronic form and in many places initiates the baby's record on a child health computer system. Births must be notified within 36 hours of occurrence.

Box 8.3: Local information systems containing data which may be available for use in an evaluation

---

Local maternity information systems

These systems are designed to record clinical information about women and their babies who are being cared for by a particular maternity unit or health service trust. Many different systems have been developed over the past twenty years. For example, up until recently, all the services in the former NW Thames Region used the St. Mary's Maternity Information system (SMMIS), a hospital-based system developed at St. Mary's Hospital, Paddington (Banfield and Beard, 1993). There are other such specialized systems such as Euroking, Stork and Protos. A few systems have been developed and used within a single hospital or area. Some of the main systems are reviewed later in this chapter. In the past some NHS regions amalgamated data from these systems into regional databases which were used for monitoring and research. With the abolition of the regional tier this no longer happens.

Hospital Patient Administration Systems (PAS)

These systems deal with hospital activity and are mainly concerned with in-patient admissions and out-patient appointments. Demographic data are collected about patients and these can be useful in describing the population being cared for.

Hospital based datasets (HBDS)

Hospital managers need to quantify the activity that takes place within each speciality in a hospital. Finance departments use this to prepare prices for care that can be quoted to purchasers. Hospital based datasets may be compiled from a maternity information system or a hospital system such as the patient administration system. They are discussed in the context of economic evaluation in Chapter 7.

Staff data and payroll data

Information on the numbers of staff employed, the hours worked and staff grade can be extracted from payroll systems.

Child health computer systems

These systems are used mainly for child health surveillance. Most are initiated by the birth notification and thus may be a useful source of maternity data. In Wales and Northern Ireland, they are the main source from which national maternity data are derived.

Child health systems are used to monitor the child's health and items of health care, as well as to invite parents to bring their child for care, notably immunizations in the early years of life. Summaries of care during delivery are usually included in a letter to the woman's GP and other health professionals. If the baby or mother dies, information can be summarized for the relevant Confidential Enquiry. A recent study of how the benefits of computerized maternity information systems could be realized identified a large range of uses to which these systems can be put (British Computer Society and NHS Executive, 1996). These are listed in Box 8.4.

Box 8.4: Possible uses for computerized maternity services information systems

Staff usage
Audit
Retrieval of statistics
Research
Print outs of summary letters, birth notifications and child health records
Initiating requests for investigations
Retrieving the results of investigations
Identifying risk factors

Management usage
Audit
Retrieval of statistics
Financial planning
Monitoring workloads

Information systems should also generate a minimum dataset for each episode of hospital inpatient care and every birth wherever it occurs. In England, if a woman gives birth during an episode of care the data are then made up of a basic dataset and a 'maternity tail' containing items specific to maternity care. The content of the current minimum dataset used in England was determined, in the mid-1980s, by the Steering Group on Health Services Information, usually known as the Körner Committee. A new minimum dataset is currently being developed. The data are aggregated nationally to form the Maternity Hospital Episode System (Maternity HES). Similar minimum datasets are used in Northern Ireland and Wales. In Wales, the data are aggregated through the Patient Episode Database for Wales (PEDW). The quality of these data is often poor. In Northern Ireland the data are aggregated through child health systems. Scotland has a much higher quality dataset collected through the SMR2 maternity discharge sheet. This has recently been revised and incorporated into the Core Patient Profile Information in Scottish Hospitals (COPPISH).

Maternity information systems or sometimes patient administration systems (PAS) can also be used to provide regular information about workload and staffing for daily management and planning purposes. Information systems should be capable of generating aggregated data in the form of statistical summaries which can be used for audit (Yudkin and Redman, 1990), evaluation and research. This was one of the features managers and midwives identified as being the most useful aspect of information systems in a recent study undertaken by the British Computer Society and NHS Executive (1996). The extent to which they are actually capable of doing this varies considerably.

Evaluating local computerized maternity information systems

The national picture

Pam Dobson, a midwife researcher with a special interest in information systems and one of the authors of this chapter, carried out a review of maternity information systems (Dobson, 1995). This review had two aims:

1. To compile a comprehensive list of existing systems in England and Wales that are used for maternity data.
2. To investigate midwives' views about these systems.

This review was necessary because an earlier survey of obstetric information systems (Yoong et al., 1993) had been aimed at obstetricians but identified midwives as the main professional group responsible for entering data. The results of Pam Dobson's review shed useful light on the picture in 1995 and thus are of relevance to midwives choosing and evaluating systems for their own units.

At the outset the midwife researcher visited maternity services where the SMMIS, Protos, Euroking and Stork systems were in use. The aim of the visits was to see what information was collected, what the methods of data input were, what uses the systems was put to and what links the system had to other systems such as the Patient Administration System. A key area of interest was the flexibility of the system. For example, could data entry fields be easily changed to facilitate the addition or removal of data items as required? Other important dimensions considered were the management of the system, the levels of interest of the various health care professionals involved, security, the monitoring of data quality and the satisfaction of the midwives using the system.

Following these preliminary visits a questionnaire was constructed and sent to the labour wards of each maternity unit in England and Wales. It was thought that if an information system was being used it would be most likely to be used on the labour ward, or people on the labour ward would know where to send the questionnaire. The questionnaire concentrated on midwifery information requirements and covered topics dealt with in the preliminary visits and with the collection of data relevant to *Changing Childbirth*, data for auditing midwifery practice, the monitoring of standards, the generation of data for compulsory returns such as CESDI and Körner, and whether the system had an ad hoc reporting facility. Other questions explored the respondents' perceptions of the advantages and disadvantages of a computer system.

The results of the survey have now been published (Dobson, 1995). Just over three quarters of Units in England and Wales responded. Figure 8.1 shows the type of computerized system in use in the 100 Units that had one. Most of the 17 Units labelled 'Others' were using adapted nursing information systems. Forty six Units reported that they were able to collect some data relevant to *Changing Childbirth*, but in 37 of these Units this was limited to data about the 'named midwife'. Seventy six Units were able to use their system to help with midwifery audit. Only 27 Units used the data they collected to monitor standards of care.

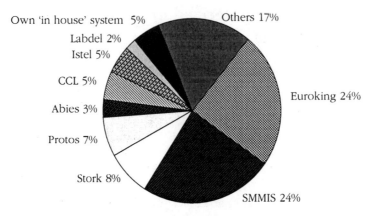

Own 'in house' system 5%
Labdel 2%
Istel 5%
CCL 5%
Abies 3%
Protos 7%
Stork 8%
Others 17%
Euroking 24%
SMMIS 24%

Fig 8.1: Computerized maternity information systems: Software used, England and Wales, 1995

Only 37 of the Units reported that they were able to change data-entry fields and of these only eight said that this could be done within six months of the request. Twenty eight Units reported that there was a midwife in post who was responsible for the management of the system, while 37 Units said that the system was managed by another professional. An area of concern was that over half the respondents reported that there was no person or policy in place to check the quality of the data in the Unit. A further ten did not know if data quality checks were carried out at all. Respondents in 40 Units were dissatisfied with the system they had and these respondents were more likely to be among those not using purpose built maternity systems.

A much more limited survey in 1996 showed some changes in the choice of system (Kenney and Macfarlane, 1996). The results of this are compared with those from earlier surveys in Table 8.1.

Computer information system	Great Britain 1992		England & Wales 1995		England & Wales 1996	
	No.	%	No.	%	No.	%
SMMIS	36	36	24	24	25	21
Euroking	13	13	24	24	24	20
Protos	–	–	7	7	11	9
Abies	–	–	3	3	3	3
Istel	6	6	5	5	2	2
CCL	13	13	5	5	7	6
Stork	–	–	8	8	14	12
Labdel	–	–	2	2	2	2
Others+	32	32	22	22	27	23
Not stated					2	2
All	100#	100	100#	100	117	100

(Source: Kenney & Macfarlane, 1996)

+ This includes own 'in house' systems

Each of these surveys obtained responses from 100 Units

Table 8.1: Type and percentage of Units using computer software

Accuracy, accessibility and relevance

One way to evaluate information systems is in terms of their accuracy, accessibility and relevance.

ACCURACY

The quality of the information collected depends on *which* data are collected and *how* they are collected. Errors can be reduced and tedious work avoided, if the maternity system is linked with other systems, so that a woman's demographic details do not have to be entered several times over. It has been shown that introducing a computer system can improve the accuracy and completeness of maternity records and reduce the time spent on record keeping (Calkin, 1994).

Accuracy and speed are possible only for people who understand the system. This depends on receiving good training. Midwives working in units with computer systems must now be trained to use them. Furthermore, the quality of the data is reduced if people are asked to collect too many items because they may become complacent and careless about the more common data items. Some systems may try to tackle this by preventing people from moving on to the next screen if the coding is not correct.

Accuracy is also likely to be improved if midwives feel they 'own' the system. It helps midwives to own the system if there is a specialist midwife to manage the system. If this midwife is also responsible for training the midwives, s/he can relate the screens to the Unit's way of working and can explain the subtleties of the coding. A computer liaison midwife can also carry out quality checks on the data collected. At King's College Hospital, the computer liaison midwife carries out monthly random checks to compare women's notes with the information entered on the computer.

Midwives are not the only people who input information about the maternity services. Clerks may have to be trained to enter and code details of surgical procedures and other obstetric outcomes in sufficient detail. For example, in one of the most commonly used coding systems, the OPCS Classification of surgical operations and procedures (OPCS, 1990), there are a number of codes for forceps delivery, codes R21.1 to R21.9, which are detailed below. These are structured in such a way that some codes are tightly defined and these are followed by broader groupings of procedures in the same category, using the abbreviation 'nec' meaning 'not elsewhere classified'.

- R21.1 – High forceps cephalic delivery with rotation
- R21.2 – High forceps cephalic delivery nec
- R21.3 – Mid forceps cephalic delivery with rotation
- R21.4 – Mid forceps cephalic delivery nec
- R21.5 – Low forceps cephalic delivery
- R21.8 – Other specified
- R21.9 – Unspecified

Information about what happens to a person during a stay in hospital is known as 'hospital based activity'. This is often assembled by coding information from manual notes or records at the end of a woman's hospital maternity care. This coded information is usually entered into the computer by clerks but it may be difficult for a clerk, or any other person who is not clinically trained, to reach decisions about how to code complex conditions. Coding will be made easier if the care givers record clinical information clearly in the records and are familiar with the basis of the coding system.

This point has been made at some length to illustrate that the information generated by computers depends on the quality of the data and on the level of expertise or training of the person putting in the data. It has to be remembered that decisions made about maternity services by hospital managers and finance directors will be based on this information. If midwife managers are to work in the best interests of the service, they need to know how the data about the service are collected, when and where coding takes place, who puts the data into the computer and who retrieves information from it. In particular, coders, who are not well trained or are unable to read poorly written notes, may have to code a forceps delivery as R21.9 unspecified, if they are unclear about exactly what happened.

Data must be as accurate as possible but they also need to be complete. Because information systems are hospital centred, data about home births and about the large amount of care provided by midwives for women who give birth at other units rarely feature in the systems. In audits, or other research projects, these data generally have to be unearthed from other, non-computerized, sources.

ACCESSIBILITY

If a system is to be 'real time', giving an instant readout, computers need to be readily accessible throughout the hospital – in the antenatal clinic, the labour ward, and in antenatal and postnatal wards. It is not practicable to have a single machine locked in a room for data to be added by one person when they have time. The computers need to be linked to a good network. To achieve up-to-date information means that some data will have to be put on by midwives, either during, or after, a contact with a pregnant woman. It is essential that the system is 'user friendly'. Many people feel defeated in front of complicated screens and assume that it is them rather than the system that is inadequate. Some systems allow data to be swiftly entered by using single keys or bar code pens. Midwives can use an open questionnaire book of bar codes scanning in the relevant code with a pen attached to the computer. In some places community midwives are beginning to use laptop computers for entering their own data away from their office. They have to understand about downloading their disks of information into the main system.

In return, for the amount of time and training midwives are being asked to invest in using information systems, they have a right to expect the system to provide them with information that is useful to them, as well as to the maternity service overall. Accuracy is also improved if the midwives can easily access the information they have collected in order to gain feedback about their work.

Information about the implementation of *Changing Childbirth* could be collected by computer provided the existing systems, with their emphasis on clinical outcomes, are modified. The data collected on the existing systems may not give the midwife any

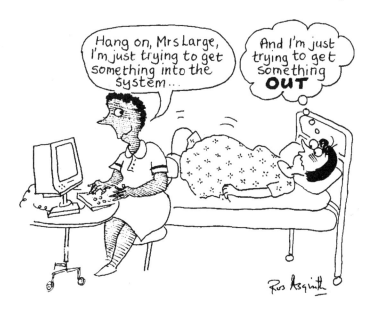

information about whether the pregnant woman had a named midwife, who was her lead professional, where she attended for antenatal check-ups, how many people she saw antenatally, whether the woman knew the person who attended her in labour, and how many people she saw postnatally. In order to obtain some of this information at present, data would have to be collected from paper records in hospital and the community and from questionnaires to women.

RELEVANCE

In some places there have been plans to use nursing information systems for maternity care. A nursing system will have one obvious inadequacy: it will not have been designed to admit one person for care and discharge two or more! A nursing system will need adapting in other ways for maternity services. This will require several levels of expertise and a lot of time to learn the system and modify it for midwives. Once this stage is reached, the supplier will have to make the necessary changes to the system or, as this has budgetary implications, the users of the system will have to try to do some modifications themselves. This will inevitably put constraints on the data to be collected. If modifications such as printing out or compiling disc files of birth notifications, or data for the Confidential Enquiry into Stillbirths and Deaths in Infancy (CESDI) are needed, then the extra work will have to be done by the supplier.

It is clear that good computerized maternity information systems, and the ability to use them, are important for all who provide and plan care, and for those evaluating a service. Computer systems have not yet caught up with some of the basic requirements in terms of data items and the need for records based on the whole childbearing episode. Most do not yet have the ability to monitor progress towards some of the objectives of *Changing Childbirth*. We would recommend that all maternity services have a midwife in post who is responsible for maternity information and probably for audit, and who has the skills, time and resources to manage this crucial area properly.

Maternity information systems are likely to become far more useful if demands are made upon them. At the same time the quality of the data is likely to improve if those who enter information get something back that is relevant to their work.

Advice about maternity information systems

If you want to find out more about current maternity information systems there are groups which can help you to start your enquiries.

- The RCOG Audit Unit in Manchester (see details in Box 9.4) will be able to put you in touch with clinicians with a special interest in maternity information systems.
- The Royal College of Midwives has a special computer interest group which should be contacted via the Education Department at the RCM.

The Changing Childbirth team should also be able to put you in touch with people interested in this.

In general it is better to get some advice from people with practical, maternity related experience of the various computer based systems before deciding to invest in one for your Unit.

References

Banfield, P.J., Beard, R.W. (1993). 'The right tool for the right job: computerised maternity data'. *MIDIRS Midwifery Digest*, Vol. 3, No. 3, p. 274.

Barron, S.L., Macfarlane, A.J. (1990). 'Collection and use of routine maternity data'. *Bailliere's Clin. Obstet. Gynaecol*, Vol. 4, pp. 681–97.

British Computer Society Nursing Specialist Group, Midwifery Focus Group and Information Management Group of the NHS Executive (1996). *Benefits Realization Monograph on Maternity Information Systems*. Leeds: NHS Executive.

Calkin, S. (1994). *An Evaluation of a Computer System Introduced into a Maternity Unit*. MSc. Thesis St Georges Hospital Medical School, London (Unpublished).

Department of Health (1997). *Hospital Delivery in England*. Statistical Bulletin (Provisional title).

Dobson, P. (1995). 'A survey of computerised midwifery information systems'. *British Journal of Midwifery*, Vol. 3, No. 9, pp. 487–490.

Information and Statistics Division (1997). *Births in Scotland 1976–1995*. Edinburgh: ISD.

Kenney, N., Macfarlane, A.D. (1996). *Use of Computerized Information Systems in Maternity Units in England and Wales: Changing Childbirth Information Survey*. Submitted for publication.

Macfarlane, A.J., Mugford, M., Johnson, A., Garcia, J. (1995). *Counting the Changes in Childbirth: Trends and Gaps in National Statistics*. Oxford: National Perinatal Epidemiology Unit.

Macfarlane, A.J., Mugford, M. (1984). *Birth Counts: Statistics of Pregnancy and Childbirth*. 2 Vols. London: HMSO.

Macfarlane, A.J. (1994a). 'Review and assessment of models of care using research, information and data: the role of routinely collected data'. In: Chamberlain, G., Patel, N. (Eds). *The Future of the Maternity Services*. London: RCOG Press. pp. 18–35.

Macfarlane, A.J. (1994b). 'Sources of data'. In: Maresh, M. (Ed). *Audit in Obstetrics and Gynaecology*. Oxford: Blackwell, pp. 18–49.

Middle, C., Macfarlane, A.J. (1995a). *Labour and Delivery in Normal Primiparous Women: Analyses of Routinely Collected Data*. Report for the Clinical Standards Advisory Group. Oxford: NPEU.

Middle, C., Macfarlane, A.J. (1995b). 'Labour and delivery of "normal" primiparous women: analysis of routinely collected data'. *British Journal of Obstetrics and Gynaecology*, Vol. 102, pp. 970–97.

ONS (1996). *Guide to Official Statistics 1996*. London: Stationery Office Edition.

Thomas, S.C. (1996). *Midwifery led Care Pilot Scheme and the MIS*. Personal communication.

Thunhurst, C., Macfarlane, A.J. (1992). 'Monitoring the health of urban populations: what statistics do we need?'. *Journal of the Royal Statistical Society,* Vol. 155, pp. 317–52.

Yoong, A., Das, S., Carroll, S., Chard, T. (1993). 'A national survey to assess current use of computerised information systems in obstetrics'. *Brit. J. Obst. Gynaec,* Vol. 100, No. 3, pp. 205–208.

Yudkin, P.L., Redman, C.W.G. (1990). 'Obstetric audit using routinely collected computerised data'. *BMJ,* Vol. 301, pp. 1371–73.

CHAPTER NINE

Evaluation Through Clinical Audit

Jo Garcia

Introduction

Although the word audit is used in a variety of ways, in this case we are using it to mean an approach that asks if agreed standards for clinical and organizational aspects of the service are being met. Audit involves setting standards, collecting data about care, providing feedback of audit results to care givers, agreeing further change, and doing another audit to see if the agreed changes are taking place. This process has been called 'the audit spiral'. Some audits only complete part of the spiral, stopping short of feedback or the repeat audit. For discussions about what is and is not audit and how it relates to topics like quality assessment see Crombie et al. (1993), Maresh (1994), Balogh (1996) and Harvey (1996).

Audit can answer questions about what is happening, but not about cause and effect. Audit is about changing care in the light of agreed standards. Some examples of audits of maternity care are given in Boxes 9.1 to 9.3.

Box 9.1: The named midwife – an audit and repeat audit

Rutherglen Maternity Hospital, Glasgow

In response to recommendations within the *Patient's Charter* the 'Named Midwife' concept was introduced in March 1994. An initial audit was carried out in June 1994 to see how well the new approach was working. This included using a short questionnaire for 100 women, a review of a sample of community midwifery records (135 records), a questionnaire for all 131 midwives and an audit of 100 records at transfer of mother and/or baby from hospital. Response rates varied. These studies provided estimates of the extent to which the targets were being achieved, and also revealed some practical problems for midwives in putting the policy into effect. Some practical recommendations were made, but no fundamental changes in the scheme introduced. A repeat audit was carried out in January 1995 using the same methods. This indicated that considerable progress had been made in implementing the changes, though there were still aspects of documentation that could be improved. The authors concluded that no major changes in the 'Named Midwife' scheme were indicated and recommended that a further audit be done in six months (Weir and Green, 1994, 1995).

This audit of an organizational change (Box 9.1) has followed the key steps in the audit cycle. The two reports are particularly useful because they discuss the views of midwives about the changes in care and also look at some of the reasons why the audit was difficult to carry out.

Box 9.2: Routine haemoglobin in the postnatal period

Derby City General Hospital

In order to look at their policies for routine haemoglobin testing, midwives in Derby carried out a retrospective audit of the casenotes of 1200 women who had given birth between January and April 1993. They found that over a third of women did not have postnatal Hb status recorded in the notes, in spite of a policy of routine testing. They also found some problems in the antenatal testing and status of women at delivery. In the light of the audit findings and other evidence, recommendations were made about testing and record keeping. In 1995 a second, smaller study was carried out which looked at one aspect of the proposed changes in policy. What would happen if selected women were tested for Hb postnatally – women with low antenatal Hb, women with an instrumental delivery and women with a blood loss of more than 500mls at delivery? A retrospective study was carried out of the records of 138 women who would not be tested under this policy (i.e. 'low risk' women). A fifth had a Hb of less than 10.5g/dcl when tested at three days after delivery, but only three of these were judged to be anaemic on the basis of more reliable tests. This suggests that testing all women at three days is not likely to be useful in detecting women who need treatment for anaemia. Following further discussion, changes in the women-held records have been made to encourage Hb testing to take place at appropriate times. It has also been agreed to try out a period of routine assessment of Hb at six days postnatal. The team are now preparing a repeat audit to assess whether their recommendations are being put into practice.

For further information about these studies contact: Maternity and Gynaecology Audit and Research, Derby City General Hospital, Uttoxeter Rd, Derby DE22 3NE.

Box 9.2 describes an audit of clinical care rather than an audit of an aspect of the organization of care. It is now part way through the audit cycle and has generated policy recommendations and a smaller research study. The next example, in Box 9.3, is an audit carried out jointly by midwives and doctors. Ideally, audit should be done by different professions in collaboration, though this may be more important for some topics than others (see a discussion in Ross, 1996).

Box 9.3: Postpartum blood loss – a multidisciplinary audit

Withington Hospital, Manchester

This audit was carried out because staff expressed concern about an apparent increase in postpartum haemorrhage. The audit was planned at a meeting of medical and midwifery staff and an audit form designed. Information was taken retrospectively from the records of 418 women who had delivered between July and September 1991. On the basis of the results, various recommendations about practice were made, for example clarification of the policy on third stage management and recommendations on operative delivery and the need to avoid delay in the repair of episiotomy. After the recommendations were circulated to staff it was agreed that a prospective audit would be carried out a year later – November 1992 to January 1993. The same data sheets were used. One finding was a marked reduction in excessive blood loss after operative delivery (Nunns et al., 1995).

Although quite a lot of audit is being done, very few reports of audits in maternity care have been published. At the end of the chapter we list various ways of getting information about audit and making contact with others who are doing audits. Publications relevant to maternity care include Maresh (1994) and Downe (1994). A useful general book is *The Audit Handbook* (Crombie et al., 1993).

Stages in the audit process

Deciding which aspects of the service to audit

In practice most clinical audits arise from a concern among staff about a particular aspect of care. There are different views about which topics should be audited. Some argue that clinical audit should be confined to topics where there is evidence about effectiveness. For example, there is poor knowledge about the effects of withholding food and drink from women in labour. If it is difficult to set standards for the audit of labour ward practice, should resources be used for audit of this aspect of care? On the other hand there is probably a need to agree working policies even though evidence is limited, and so some monitoring of the policies may be justified. Perhaps the availability of evidence about a particular aspect of care should increase the priority given to it in decisions about what to audit (Grimshaw and Russell, 1993; Baker and Fraser, 1995). In addition, even in clinical audits, there are questions about the organizational aspects of the service – availability of records, missing samples or tests results, duplication of work – and these may be usefully audited.

Setting standards

Standards are set in clinical practice by using reliable evidence about effectiveness combined with best estimates on the basis of limited evidence and, least usefully, accepted but unexamined ways of doing things. In addition, as mentioned above, policies for care often include organizational recommendations that are aimed to improve efficiency. One approach to standard setting in midwifery care is represented by *Midwifery Monitor* (Hughes and Goldstone, 1993) which was developed from nursing quality models. It aims to set detailed standards for various aspects of midwifery work. It has been used quite widely in evaluations, but these have rarely been the subject of published reports. An exception is the evaluation of One-to-One midwifery at Queen Charlotte's which included an audit based on Midwifery Monitor (McCourt and Page, 1996). In nursing there has been an emphasis on the involvement of clinical nurses in the development of standards for care that can be assessed in audit (see for example, Royal College of Nursing, 1990; Harvey, 1996). The idea that standards should be based on evidence is relatively new, and so there is a need for some rethinking about approaches to audit in all specialties.

Moving to auditable objectives

Next, the standards usually need to be translated into detailed objectives that can be audited. For example, a common goal is to improve continuity of carer, and this can be measured by looking at issues like the proportion of women that are cared for in labour by a midwife from the woman's team, or the proportion of women who know the midwife who cares for them in labour. The move from general goals to auditable aspects of care is a crucial part of the process because it is about practical aspects of care, and about what can actually be measured (Baker and Fraser, 1995).

Getting the information you need

The next step is to work out how to get the information needed and again this is important because it depends on the human and financial resources available to the project. If available, local sources of routinely collected information can contribute to this process. Local maternity information systems can provide material for audit so that midwives have less extra form-filling to do. In practice though, they are often not flexible enough to answer the sort of questions that are being posed about care in the light of *Changing Childbirth* (see the chapter on information in maternity care). If data need to be collected specially for the audit, then time and care need to go into the design of the forms or data entry modules, and the decisions about sample size (see Maresh, 1994). You may want to ask for advice from an audit department or other experienced researchers at this point. It is frustrating to put time and effort into an audit only to find out that too few cases were included, or a vital piece of information was missed.

Extracting data from hospital records retrospectively is time consuming, but this is often the only way to get the information you need (see Chapter 7 for more on this). An alternative is to add a special form to the records to collect the extra information prospectively (i.e. at the time that care is being given). This is more likely to be successful if the staff who are asked to fill in the forms are interested in the audit. This is true of the whole process – staff involvement in setting the topics for audit and working out the best way to get the data should help to make the audit successful.

Feeding back the results

Once information is collected and analysed it should be fed back as promptly as possible to those concerned with the care, or with the data collection. The goal should be to set up audit as an ongoing process of information feedback, so that care givers know what is happening with the care they provide. If the audit indicates that change is needed then an agreement should be reached about how to make the changes. Plans should be made for a follow-up audit to see what has happened.

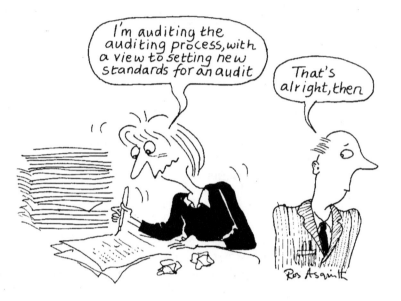

Writing up the results

It is very useful to have an audit project written up, and if possible published, so that others can benefit from the experience. In maternity care the new audit advice services and databases should be very helpful (see Box 9.4).

Audit is a key part of the assessment of different patterns of care. It *is* limited in what it can do, but it is relatively cheap, especially if routine maternity data can be used. When changes are being made to the way that care is organized, it is crucial to set objectives for the service and to look to see if those objectives are met. It cannot be assumed that changes will always have the effects expected. If a new scheme is supposed to improve continuity of carer, we need to set detailed objectives and then look to see, for example, how many women are visited at home by three or more community midwives, or how many staff are present at delivery. Prompt feedback of accurate and relevant information to care givers should be a vital part of improving care.

Box 9.4: Sources of advice on maternity audit

There are very few published guides for maternity care to help with any of these steps in the audit process. In the mean time we would advise people to start out by contacting anyone in their local area responsible for audit (medical, nursing or clinical).

There are also some national sources of advice that are either available now, or planned to start soon. These are:

- The National Centre for Clinical Audit. This is being set up by a consortium of 14 health care organizations and will be based at the British Medical Association. The aim is to ensure that existing and future audit projects, whether national, regional or local, are fully informed about similar or related projects. For more information contact the Centre on 0171 383 6451.

- The Midwifery and Nursing Audit Information Service. This is a joint project of the Royal College of Midwives and Royal College of Nursing and is funded by the Department of Health. Written queries should be addressed to the RCM Midwifery Audit Co-ordinator, RCM Headquarters, 15 Mansfield Street, London W1M 0BE. For telephone enquiries contact the Audit Information Office, Royal College of Nursing, 20 Cavendish Square, London W1M 0AB – 0171 629 7464. The project includes a database of midwifery and nursing audit, which may be useful for making contact with those working on similar topics or at local hospitals.

- The Royal College of Obstetricians and Gynaecologists Audit Unit. This is based at St Mary's Hospital, Hathersage Rd, Manchester M13 0JH, 0161 276 6300. This Unit welcomes enquiries about all types of maternity audit, including midwifery and community based care, and will give advice and put people in touch with those doing similar projects. Two midwives are currently working there. It has a database of over 5000 maternity audits, including protocols.

Putting your project on a database means that other people can build on your work. If it is an audit project then contact the National Centre for Clinical Audit, the RCOG Audit Unit or the RCM Midwifery Audit Co-ordinator (see above). Research projects in midwifery should be registered with MIRIAD at Midwifery Studies, 22 Hyde Terrace, Leeds LS2 9LN. If in doubt about whether your work is research or audit, write for advice.

References

Baker, R., Fraser, R.C. (1995). 'Development of review criteria: linking guidelines and assessment of quality'. *British Medical Journal,* Vol. 311, pp. 370–373.

Balogh, R. (1996). 'Exploring the links between audit and the research process'. *Nurse Researcher,* Vol. 3, pp. 5–16.

Crombie, I.K., Davies, H.T.O., Abraham, S.C.S., Florey, C.V. (1993). *The Audit Handbook.* Chichester: John Wiley.

Downe, S. (1994). 'Maternity audit in practice'. *British Journal of Midwifery,* Vol. 2, pp. 77–82.

Grimshaw, J.M., Russell, I.T. (1993). 'Achieving health gain through clinical guidelines. I Developing scientifically valid guidelines'. *Quality in Health Care,* Vol. 2, pp. 243–48.

Harvey, G. (1996). 'Relating quality assurance and audit to the research process in nursing'. *Nurse Researcher,* Vol. 3, pp. 35–46.

Hughes, D.J.F., Goldstone, L.A. (1993). *Midwifery Monitor.* Loughton, Essex: Gale Centre Publications.

McCourt, C., Page, L. (Eds.) (1996*). Report on the Evaluation of One-to-One Midwifery.* Thames Valley University and The Hammersmith Hospitals Trust.

Maresh, M. (1994). *Audit in Obstetrics and Gynaecology.* Oxford: Blackwells Scientific.

Nunns, D., Dewart, P.J., Hirsch, P.J., Elstein, M. (1995). 'Postpartum blood loss: implementation of recommendations following a retrospective audit resulting in improved patient care'. *Journal of Obstetrics and Gynaecology,* Vol. 15, pp. 230–232.

Ross, F. (1996). 'Interprofessional audit: the need for teamwork when researching quality of care'. *Nurse Researcher,* Vol. 3, pp. 47–57.

Royal College of Nursing (1990). *Quality Patient Care: the Dynamic Standard Setting System.* Harrow: Scutari.

Weir, C.L., Green, E. (1994). *The Named Midwife Thus Far: An Evaluation.* Glasgow: Victoria Infirmary NHS Trust.

Weir, C.L., Green, E. (1995). *The Named Midwife, Another Look: An Evaluation.* Glasgow: Victoria Infirmary NHS Trust.

Further reading

Ball, J.A., Hughes, D. (1994). 'Quality assurance in maternity care'. In: Bennet, R., Brown, L. (Eds). *Myles Textbook for Midwives.* 12th edition. Edinburgh: Churchill Livingstone.

Ball, J.A. (1993). 'Workload measurement in midwifery'. In: Alexander, J., Levy, V., Roche, S. (Eds). *Midwifery Practice: A Research Based Approach.* Basingstoke: Macmillan.

Ball, J.A., Washbrook, M. (1996). *Birthrate Plus: A Framework for Workforce Planning and Decision-Making for Midwifery Services.* Hale, Cheshire: Books for Midwives Press.

Crombie, I.K., Davies, H.T.O. (1996). *Research in Health Care: Design, Conduct and Interpretation of Health Services Research.* Chichester: Wiley.

Paterson, C.M., Chappel, J.C., Beard, R.W., Joffe, M., Steer, P.J., Wright, C.S.W. (1991). 'Evaluating the quality of the maternity services – a discussion paper'. *British Journal of Obstetrics and Gynaecology,* Vol. 98, pp. 1073–1078.

CHAPTER TEN

Planning An Evaluation: Bibliographic, Financial and Human Resources

Jane Sandall

The purpose of this chapter is to review the practical steps which need to be taken before starting an evaluation. This chapter deals with three main topics:

- how to find out what work, if any, has already been done
- how to get financial support
- how to get access and ethical approval.

Evaluations can differ in scale, from a simple audit to a comprehensive evaluation of all aspects of a particular service. It is therefore important to ensure that the amount of preliminary work is consistent with the overall scale of the evaluation. This chapter attempts to provide some guidance on this as well as indicating what work you will have to do yourself, what you might be able to get help with and from whom that help might be forthcoming. Addresses and telephone numbers of the many organizations and services mentioned in this chapter can be found in a series of tables (see Appendix).

Finding out what has been done before and what work is ongoing

Finding out about other research and evaluation on your topic of interest involves searching both the published literature and databases which contain information about work in progress. It may also involve contacting national organizations which have been set up to support and monitor research and evaluation activity (see Table 1 of the Appendix for further details).

There is much to be gained from reviewing other work before starting your own. Most importantly, it can indicate what is already known and so prevent endless re-discovery of the wheel. In addition, it can point out areas that need further study, show you where potential pitfalls and difficulties may lie, indicate what research methods may be best and provide some kind of yardstick against which to measure your own endeavour. A recent guide to sources of research-based information on maternity care is a useful starting point (National Childbirth Trust, 1995).

If you are clear from the outset that you only want to undertake a very small scale evaluation, or are concerned with the local implementation of a well tried and tested scheme, then a detailed literature search is probably not necessary and may use up time which might be better spent on the evaluation itself. At the other end of the spectrum you may be interested in undertaking a systematic review of all the research evidence relating to, for example, team midwifery as a method of improving continuity of carer, before you introduce a system of team midwifery which you then plan to evaluate. As part of a drive to make health care evidence-based rather than driven by custom and practice, and make research more focused on what is not known, systematic reviewing of the literature has become a method of research in its own right. A number of centres, of which the Cochrane Collaboration is perhaps the best known, have been set up both in the United Kingdom and throughout the world to co-ordinate this kind of activity. Details of these organizations can be found in Tables 1 and 3 of the Appendix.

Searching the literature

It is a good idea to try and find out what library resources are available to you. Ideally you will want to use a specialist health or medical library. Postgraduate centres in NHS Trusts often have such libraries as do universities and colleges which undertake training of midwifery, medical, nursing and paramedical staff. Membership of professional organizations may provide you with some kind of library service. MIDIRS (Midwives Information and Resource Service) also provides bibliographic services which are mentioned in more detail later.

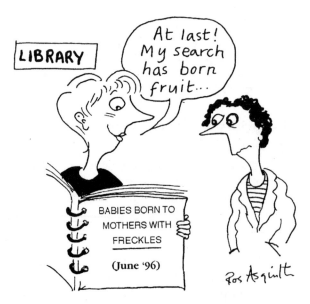

If you have never undertaken a formal literature search before, find a suitable library and ask a librarian for help. If you are going to be searching electronically (i.e. using a computer to gain access to databases) you will need help with this if you haven't done it before. It can be quite costly and some libraries will do it for you and charge you. You will also have to pay for copies of the articles that you ask for as a result of the searches, and this can be expensive if you are doing a large literature review.

Doing the search

Before doing a literature search you need to have a reasonably clear idea of what your topic of interest is. It is helpful to draw up a list of the key words and phrases that might help identify your area of interest. Most of the tools devised to assist with the search of existing information usually do so on the basis of key words. If you were interested in evaluations of team midwifery, then your list of key words might include EVALUATION, TEAM MIDWIFERY, CONTINUITY OF CARE, MIDWIFE AUTONOMY. If you just searched on a general term such as EVALUATION you could find thousands of references. Key words like this should only be used in combination with other relevant terms and thus you may need to refine your search as it progresses. When planning a search the following guidelines may prove helpful (adapted from Jadad and McQuay, 1993).

* A search takes time
* Be systematic
* Acquire some background knowledge
* Keep an outline of your research design to hand
* When in doubt, include
* Save your search strategy for possible reuse.

As reviews are a crucial part of transferring research into practice and guiding the planning of new work, it is important that they are done well and systematically. For a substantial review of the literature it is best to write down what your methods are and to document all the steps you take in looking for literature. Part of this is saving your search strategy when using electronic databases, so you know what you did and can repeat it.

Special databases of references, such as MEDLINE, have been developed to assist with literature searching. These are essentially just lists of journal articles, often including the abstract (a summary) sorted by subject or author. The organizations which maintain these indexes will scan a defined group of journals so it is useful to be aware of possible gaps in their coverage. For example, they may only include journals from certain countries or miss certain titles or subject areas. These indexes are published in either paper or electronic forms and sometimes both. Box 10.1 lists some of the main paper indexes and abstracting journals which can assist a manual search and Box 10.2 gives details of some of the main electronic tools.

Box 10.1: Indexes, abstracting journals and bibliographies published on paper for manual searching

Indexing journals

Publish a systematic list of bibliographic references for journal articles, grouped under subject headings. They give no information about the content of the article, but are produced quickly. Some examples are CINAHL and Index Medicus (see Appendix).

Abstracting journals

Publish references and abstracts from journals, for example, Nursing Research Abstracts. They are not as up to date as the indexing journals or on-line databases.

Citation indexes

These are compiled from reference lists of published articles, for example, the Social Science Citation Index. They are arranged alphabetically by author, with details of articles they have written which have then been referred to by other authors. Thus, a seminal article, such as Flint, C., Poulengeris, P., Grant, A. (1989). 'The 'know your midwife' scheme – a randomized controlled trial of continuity of care by a team of midwives'. *Midwifery*, 5:11–16, will be cited by many other authors. This is a useful way of finding key papers in the area you are interested in.

Bibliographies

Whitakers Books in Print covers books in print and on sale in the UK (also *Books in Print* for USA) but not all publishers are represented. For example, material published by research institutes and organizations such as the King's Fund are not listed. HMSO publishes its own catalogue of materials in print, but some departments, including the Department of Health, publish separately and should be listed in British Official Publications not published by HMSO. The British National Bibliography lists all the monographs published within Britain and is based on the stock of the British Library. The American equivalent is the Catalogue of the Library of Congress.

Reports, conferences and theses (grey literature) are very difficult to trace after publication. The British Reports, Translations and Theses (BRTT) published by the British Library every month lists reports, theses and translations produced by Government organizations, industry, universities and HMSO. It is divided into topic sections, for example, humanities, psychology, medical sciences and social sciences.

These directories should be available in a large university library. For a list of specialist libraries see Directory of Medical and Health Care Libraries in the UK and Republic of Ireland.

Box 10.2: Electronic literature searching

CD ROM

These days the best way to start a literature search is to use the CD ROM and computer databases (see Appendix). The most widely available source is MEDLINE. Other databases may carry a charge and be expensive. Searches can be either printed out or downloaded onto a floppy disc.

Internet resources

The Internet is a huge network of computers that spans the globe. It is used by institutions such as government departments, universities, hospitals, schools and the general public (see Millman et al., 1995). It can be used to search for information, for example, the Midwifery Internet Resource is at Birmingham University (see Appendix) and contains information about other midwifery resources on the Internet world-wide (Anthony, 1996). Through the Internet it is possible to access MEDLINE, the Cochrane Collaboration, *Encyclopaedia Britannica* and increasingly some electronic journals, i.e. the BMJ went on-line in May 1995 and users are able to browse and download structured abstracts and the full text of some papers. Discussion lists also exist (see Appendix) whose aim is usually to discuss new ideas, research, events, education and grants in particular areas of interest (Delamothe, 1995; Millman et al., 1995).

On line

Many university and other specialist health service libraries have their catalogues on computer and these can be searched for books and reports. They may also be a good place to locate reports on work done locally which may have never been formally published. On-line searches are now available through the Internet. All universities are connected and staff and students have free access to, for example, BIDS (see Table 1 of the Appendix). Some Trusts and health authorities are networked but may only give restricted access (see Lee and Millman, 1995; Rowlands et al., 1995).

MIDIRS undertakes literature searches of their own database of publications relevant to midwifery which contains information based on scans of 550 journals and goes back to 1986. They have over 300 standard searches which, at the time of writing, cost £4.20 for UK subscribers to MIDIRS digest and £10.50 to other people. They will also undertake individualized searches for £5.95 for subscribers and £15.00 for others. Discounted rates are available to students.

As compilation of these indexes takes time, there are a number of current awareness services available. Midwives Information and Resource Service (MIDIRS) produces a digest with original articles and summaries of relevant books or papers published elsewhere and *Current Contents* reproduces the title pages of journals in each specialty (for further details of these see Tables 2 and 3 of the Appendix to this chapter).

Finding out about research in progress

If a project is in progress then it is unlikely for anything to have been published. Box 10.3 lists compendia which include research and evaluation of maternity care. It is important to draw upon existing networks such as the Changing Childbirth Team contacts register and the RCM Changing Childbirth Special Interest Group to find out about research and practice initiatives in progress (see Table 3 of the Appendix). Chapter 9 *Evaluation Through Clinical Audit* also contains the names and addresses of national organizations which co-ordinate and support audit work. Most researchers are happy to talk about pitfalls and problems that they have encountered by phone but these difficulties tend to get glossed over when the findings are written up.

Box 10.3: Compendia of research in progress

- Nursing Research Abstracts
- Current Research in Britain (British Library Publication)
- MIRIAD – a register of completed and ongoing research in midwifery in Britain is held at Leeds University
- English National Board has compiled a Health Care Database (see Appendix)
- The National Research Register contains ongoing and planned research supported by the NHS
- Details of ongoing projects funded by NHS Research and Development money can be found in Research and Development: Towards an evidence-based health service (Department of Health, 1995).

Reviewing and analysing the results of your search

There are now several texts on reading a research article critically, (for example Milne and Chambers, 1993), appraising the literature as a whole (Cullum, 1994; Sheldon et al., 1993) and appraising reviews of the literature (Oxman and Guyatt, 1988; Oxman, 1994). One of the key messages is to be clear about your criteria for judging the research you read, and for including or excluding studies in a review. Someone who reads your review should be able to copy what you did.

Obtaining financial resources for an evaluation

If your planned evaluation is an audit, then it may be possible to do this within existing NHS resources. If you work for an NHS Trust then they may well have a clinical audit office who can help. If you are undertaking an evaluation as part of work for a qualification or as part of your salaried post, then you may be the only resource the evaluation needs and hence applying for funding would only be appropriate if additional money was needed to cover the costs of services such as printing or postage, which might not be available to you. If, however, your evaluation is going to require additional staff or other resources, then you will need to apply for funding. For those who work in the NHS, individual Trusts may have funds available and there may be someone who has a research and development support role who can provide help and advice. The most likely port of call, however, will be the NHS Research and Development programme. This is operated on a regional basis within a national strategic framework.

Within England, some regional arms of the NHS Executive (formerly Regional Health Authorities) have special responsibility for a national programme of research, in a particular area, on behalf of NHS Executive. For example, South Thames NHS Executive recently completed a competition for funding research on priority topics within the maternal and child health field. At the time of writing it is not clear whether any more research funding will be available within this specific programme. Each regional office also commissions research of relevance to that region, has a 'responsive' funding programme to which proposals can be submitted and has funds for research training. As these operate in slightly different ways in each region, you need to find out exactly what is available in your region. For example, the South West NHS Executive has a project grants scheme for 'Developments in the organization of care' which is specifically aimed at promoting 'a critical and evaluative approach to organizational development by all health professionals' (NHS Executive South and West, 1996). Each region has a Regional Director of Research and Development, a Research and Development manager and support staff. Enquiries should therefore be directed to the Regional Research and Development office. If you have access to the Internet, further details of Regional Offices can be found by going through the home page of the Department of Health (see Table 4 of the Appendix).

The situation is similar but different in Northern Ireland, Scotland and Wales. It is best to check with the offices responsible for NHS Research and Development in each of these countries to find out exactly what funding is available and how you apply for it.

Other potential major funders are listed in Box 10.4. It should be noted that most of these organizations fund research. Thus, your proposed evaluation would have to demonstrate clearly that it would add to knowledge rather than simply indicate whether a particular way of organizing maternity care worked locally. In addition to major funding agencies, smaller institutions such as charities and trusts also have funds. Lists of directories which contain further information on these can be found in Box 10.5.

Box 10.4: Potential source of financial support for evaluations

Within the NHS
District and Trust sources
NHS Research and Development programme

Funding Councils
Economic and Social Research Council (ESRC)
Medical Research Council (MRC)

Medical and other charities
Of particular relevance: Wellbeing – Royal College of Obstetricians & Gynaecologists
Iolanthe Midwifery Trust
Nuffield Foundation
Wellcome Foundation

Occasionally you will also see advertisements from various bodies (for example Leverhume, Churchill Fellowships, Harkness Foundation) seeking research proposals or offering research fellowships, sometimes around particular themes. These adverts may appear in medical and health journals as well as in national broadsheet newspapers.

Box 10.5: Directories of charities and other trusts who fund research

---

Booth, J.D.L. (1997). *Directory of Grant Making Trusts*. London: Charities Aid Foundation.

Fitzherbert, L., Eastwood, M.A. (1997). *Guide to Major Trusts*. London: Directory of Social Change.

National Institute for Nursing (1995). *Directory of Funding for Nurses*. Oxford: National Institute for Nursing.

Preparing a protocol

It is essential to prepare a detailed plan or protocol before starting your evaluation, no matter how small it is, and even if you do not plan to apply for funding for it. A protocol sets out the exact nature of what is to be investigated and a detailed account of the methods. It is important to think this all through carefully before you begin work. You will need this if your evaluation has to be submitted to a research ethics committee and if you are applying for funding, you will also have to submit detailed plans of your proposed work, usually on a special form supplied by the funding agency. Having a detailed research plan that is agreed and approved by everyone involved at the outset can prevent disagreements later. Box 10.6 indicates the sections that a protocol should normally contain.

Box 10.6: Sections of a protocol

Title

Purpose or rationale for the evaluation

Background
This should give the context in which the evaluation is to be set and include a preliminary review of relevant literature.

Aims and objectives
The key question or questions which the evaluation will address should be included here together with details of the anticipated outcome from the evaluation.

Details of the method or methods of evaluation

Sample
Including details of access and confidentiality.

Methods of data collection and analysis
This should include details of any standard questionnaires which may be used and how the data are to be processed including quality control procedures. Details are required for both quantitative and qualitative evaluation.

Timeplan
This should include the time from the literature review through to the preparation of a final report. Including a diagram indicating how many weeks or months each aspect of the evaluation will take is useful. Remember to allow time for holidays.

Details of the evaluation
Names of those who will be involved in the evaluation with allocated roles and responsibilities.

If you are using this protocol to apply for funding then it will also need to include:

Detailed justification for support and costings
These should include estimated costs of all resources required: people's time and skill level, clerical and technical support, equipment, training and consumables.

Curriculum Vitae of proposers

If you are applying formally for research funding then details are given in Box 10.7 of how to cost your proposal. Proposals submitted to funding agencies will be sent out to anonymous referees for assessment. Referees will know who the applicants are.

Box 10.7: Costing a research proposal

Decide early who will do the work. The application should state the allocation of time and responsibilities for carrying out and writing up the research of each member of the team. Conditions of service (British Sociological Association (BSA), 1994) and guidelines of professional conduct (BSA, 1993) need to be clearly stated.

You need to justify and cost any specialist help you need. Many projects will also need clerical help and you have to decide whether to employ someone or employ casual help, for example, for the typing up of interview transcripts.

An accurate budget is vital and advice can be obtained from the funding bodies, finance officers in host institutions and other experienced researchers. You also need to check if you can transfer money between categories in the budget and from year to year in the project.

General points to check

Conferences – Check whether funders allow attendance. Some will allow attendance where papers are being given (one per year/team member is a reasonable estimate).

Data processing – Can either be done by members of the research team or commercial services. It's important to check what sort of quality control procedures commercial services use.

Equipment – It is usually assumed that you will have most of the basic equipment that you need (such as a desk, filing cabinet etc). Sometimes equipment such as transcribers (playback machines for taped recordings which permit the playback speed to be slowed so that the speech can be written or typed out) can be purchased.

Host institution – Most universities have a section responsible for research proposals. It is important to contact them early and enlist their help. The quality of these services varies.

Overheads – Increasingly overheads such as heat, light and space are being charged to funders. You will need to check your institution's policy. The rates charged are usually a percentage of the total grant. These rates can vary greatly from a low rate of 20 per cent to over 100 per cent.

Post project publication costs – Needs to be considered. Ask for what you need for dissemination.

Salaries – In most organizations there are agreed salary scales. In addition, it is important to allow for annual increments, superannuation and national insurance. You will also need to take advice on employment legislation.

Recurrent costs – Most grants only cover costs specific to research and you need to check what proportion is carried by host institutions e.g. phone and photocopying costs.

Travel – Costs should include pilot interviews, access visits and visits to libraries in other institutions (inter library loans may also have to be paid for). Check policies and rates with your institution.

In funded research, one person is usually designated the Principal Investigator, responsible for the scientific and fiscal conduct of the research (see Box 10.8). Many institutions have requirements about who may take this role – for example, only a tenured faculty member, department head or dean. Conflict can occur when the true 'owner' of the project does not have this title. It is important to clarify who owns the data; is it the funding body, the institution doing the research or the researchers? Publication credit is also subject to institutional rules. It is wise to agree, in writing, how matters relating to publication will be handled. Who will write the first draft, who else will be an author, who expects to see material prior to publication and what right of veto they possess, all needs to be agreed.

Box 10.8: Responsibilities of the principal investigator

- Managing the research monies
- Evaluation meets ethical obligations
- Rigorous conduct of evaluation
- Ensuring completion
- Dissemination of findings

Research ethics committees

A research proposal must be submitted to the local research ethics committee if the research work involves people. The existence of unethical practice in health research is still highlighted by user groups (Consumers for Ethics in Research, 1994) despite the codes and guidelines (Department of Health, 1991). Research ethics committees were set up originally in Britain to consider clinical research and are now dealing with health services and social research. Different committees apply very different policies, a fact which causes major problems for multicentre trials and national surveys. For example, a recent review (Alberti, 1995) states that not all committees required consent forms, and the response time varied from 6 to 161 days. Further problems identified were that dominant personalities biased committees, and doubt was expressed about whether they had adequate expertise to assess applications (particularly qualitative methodologies and complex statistical studies). If your evaluation consists of an audit only, then it may not need to go to a research ethics committee for approval. Seek advice locally on this. There are moves to set up regionally based committees which would review applications where the research is to be undertaken in a number of centres.

It is essential to plan well in advance for ethical approval. Research based in higher education often has to undergo additional ethical review from a university committee and this may only sit once or twice a term. Local NHS ethics committees often have deadlines for applications that only occur every two to three months and if the committee is busy, your application may not be processed at that meeting. The protocol needs to be presented along with sample information sheets for staff and users and sample consent forms. If more than one committee is being approached, it is essential to be systematic and organized and it is advisable to talk to the secretary of each committee to check whether an application is needed and to obtain application guidelines. It is worth enquiring if you also need to be prepared to support your application in person and to allow expenses relating to gaining ethical approval in your budget. Log all phone calls made in connection with this and keep correspondence carefully.

Expert help

If you need statistical or epidemiological expertise, then it is important to consult the relevant person at the beginning to decide what type and level of involvement is needed. This is because you need to decide on your analysis before you collect the data. You need to work out whether it is advice you need, or for a statistician or epidemiologist to be involved and undertake some of the work. If it is the latter then you need to consider who is going to do this, and the cost involved. It is also important to select the person carefully. You want someone who is familiar with the type of data you intend to collect and the methods you are using. It is important to be able to communicate with them; if they are consistently talking at a level you don't understand, it is not your fault. You must be assertive and ask for clarification. They should be able to work at your level and deliver and explain findings in a way you understand. There are other experts – economists, health service researchers, psychologists or computer programmers – who you may also need to consult. Choose your expert carefully. An impressive sounding job title is not a guarantee of real expertise. Always ask for concrete evidence of their past work and talk to people with whom they have worked in the past to find out how useful they found a particular expert.

For those based in the NHS it can be advantageous to link up with higher education because this may provide access to an extensive library, computer hardware and software resources and access to expert help. This may be in the form of collaborative teams, consultancies or commonly for the researcher to register for part time study on a research methods course. It is also important to bear in mind that those working in higher education, who might be engaged as consultants to a project, may be required by their employers to charge for their time. It is as well to be aware that academics are under considerable pressure to attract research funding and to publish. Thus, their agenda, or that of their employers, may be different from yours.

The politics of evaluations

It is almost inevitable that evaluations will have political dimensions. New approaches to care will have their sponsors and critics. Staff running programmes will have a lot to gain or lose from the outcomes of an evaluation. This guarantees that whatever the results of the evaluation, some will be pleased and others not. The evaluator may be open to criticism either on methodological grounds or political grounds or the latter masquerading as the former. The main implication of this is that it pays to give meticulous attention to design and conduct of the study and to ensure that the legitimate concerns of all those involved have been taken into account.

Before data collection starts, all those upon whom co-operation depends must understand the project and have given it their support. Developing the protocol with their help is a very useful way of initiating this process. It can be helpful to draw up a list of all the people who may need to be informed: a list of such people is given in Box 10.9.

> **Box 10.9:** People whose support may have to be enlisted before a research project begins
>
> - Trust chief executive and senior managers
> - Research ethics committee
> - Clinical director and relevant consultants
> - Director of midwifery services and midwifery staff
> - Medical records officer
> - Clinic clerks
> - Local medical committee
> - General practitioners
> - Professional organizations/trade union representatives
> - User group representatives
> - Maternity Services Liaison Committee.

Overcoming difficulties

Concerns with time and confidentiality are common reasons for reluctant co-operation, particularly when Trusts feel information may be sensitive. Such concerns need to be addressed actively, for example, by suggesting that interviews are held in lunch periods, or evenings with the permission of those involved. Emphasize that non-participant observation will not interfere with work and ensure that it does not in practice. The concern with confidentiality can be addressed by suggesting that a report of the study will come to the organization first to identify sensitive information. On the other hand, clear agreement needs to be established from the start about the power of veto of the organization being studied, to avoid findings being suppressed. It is important, though, that everyone involved in a project is aware of confidentiality issues.

Conflicts of interest

Health professionals who have been active in the development of a new service and also seek to evaluate it may face conflicts. As insiders they need to step back and view the service as objectively as they can. The disadvantages of being an insider may vary with the methodology being used. In ethnographic research, people will continue to relate to you in your old role and you may miss commonplace events. Colleagues may be unwilling to be observed by another colleague and respondents to in-depth interviewing may be reluctant to open up to you, particularly if you have had a managerial role. On the other hand you will have excellent knowledge of the organization and an insight into crucial issues. If you are involved in administering anonymous questionnaires or in randomized trials, then there is still the possibility that your involvement in the service could compromise your objectivity, or that others may think that it has.

These inherent conflicts between the role of clinician and evaluator may be minimized by the strategies suggested in Box 10.10.

Box 10.10: Strategies for minimizing conflict between roles as clinician and evaluator

---

- Try to foresee conflicts that may arise in the study, for example, ethnographic research in midwifery has led to dilemmas for researchers when bad practice is observed (Hunt and Symonds, 1995).

- Make a plan for dealing with any possible conflicts.

- Record responses to such situations so that you can examine the data later when reviewing the impact of your role as researcher on the data generated.

- Collaborate with experienced researchers.

- Your natural tendency will be to adopt the clinician role with clients rather than a researcher role. If possible use someone without clinical experience or from outside the study site to collect the data and interact with clients.

Research has many political and ethical aspects that are not necessarily covered in detail by research ethics committees. Confidentiality and honesty need to be considered at all stages of a project. Good, thoughtful and well managed research is more ethical and more useful because it is less likely to lead to misleading results and waste people's time. An example of attempts to balance the rights and responsibilities of researchers can be seen in the British Sociological Association's Statement of Ethical Practice (1992) and the British Psychological Society guidelines (1991). They address relationships with research participants, sponsors and funders, covert research, anonymity, confidentiality and privacy.

References

Alberti, K.G. (1995). 'Local research ethics committees'. *British Medical Journal,* Vol. 311, pp. 639–641.

Anthony, D. (1996). 'Midwifery resources on the Internet'. *British Journal of Midwifery,* Vol. 4, pp. 645–652.

British Psychological Society (1991). *Code of Conduct, Ethical Principles and Guidelines.* Leicester: BPS.

British Sociological Association (1992). *Statement of Ethical Practice.* Durham: BSA.

British Sociological Association (1993). *Guidelines for Professional Conduct.* Durham: BSA.

British Sociological Association (1994). *Guidelines on Applications for Research Funding.* Durham: BSA.

Consumers for Ethics in Research (1994). *Spreading the Word on Research.* London: CERES.

Cullum, N. (1994). 'Critical review of the literature'. In: Hardey, M., Mulhall, A. (Eds). *Nursing Research: Theory and Practice.* London: Chapman Hall.

Delamothe, T. (1995). 'British Medical Journal on the Internet'. *British Medical Journal,* Vol. 310, pp. 1343–1344.

Department of Health (1991). *Local Research Ethics Committees.* London: DH.

Department of Health (1995). *Research and Development: Towards an Evidence Based Health Service.* London: DH.

Hunt, S., Symonds, A. (1995). *The Social Meaning of Midwifery*. Basingstoke: Macmillan.

Jadad, A.R., McQuay, H.J. (1993). 'Be systematic in your searching'. *British Medical Journal*, Vol. 307, pp. 66–68.

Lee, N., Millman, A. (1995). 'Linking your computer to the outside world'. *British Medical Journal*, Vol. 311, pp. 381–384.

Millman, A., Lee, N., Kealy, K. (1995). 'The Internet'. *British Medical Journal*, Vol. 311, pp. 440–443.

Milne, R., Chambers, L. (1993). 'How to read a research article critically'. *Health Libraries Review*, Vol. 10, p. 39.

National Childbirth Trust (1995). *Through the Maze: A Guide to Sources of Research Based Information on Pregnancy, Birth and Postnatal Care*. London: National Childbirth Trust & King's Fund.

NHS Executive South and West (1996). *Research and Development Project Grants*. Guidance for Research Support.

Oxman, A.D. (1994). 'Checklists for review articles'. *British Medical Journal*, Vol. 309, pp. 648–651.

Oxman, A.D., Guyatt, G.H. (1988). 'Guidelines for reading literature reviews'. *Canadian Medical Association Journal*, Vol. 138, pp. 697–703.

Rowlands, J., Morrow, T., Lee, N., Millman, N. (1995). 'Online searching'. *British Medical Journal*, Vol. 311, pp. 500–504.

Sheldon, T.A., Song, F., Davey Smith, G. (1993). 'Critical appraisal of the medical literature: How to assess whether health care interventions do more harm than good'. In: Drummond, M.F., Maynard, A. (Eds). *Purchasing and Providing Cost-Effective Health Care*. Edinburgh: Churchill-Livingstone.

Further reading

Booth, A. (1995). *The Scharr Guide to Evidence Based Practice*. SCHARR Information Resources, University of Sheffield, 30 Regent Street, Sheffield, S1 4DA.

Crombie, I.K. (1996). *The Pocket Guide to Critical Appraisal*. London: BMJ Publishing.

Data Protection Registrar (1989). *Guide to the Data Protection Act. Volume 1–8*. Office of the Data Protection Registrar, Springfield House, Water Lane, Wilmslow, Cheshire, SK9 5AX.

Department of Health (1993). *Research for Health*. London: DH.

Department of Health (1993). *Report of the Taskforce on the Strategy for Research in Nursing, Midwifery and Health Visiting*. London: DH.

Department of Health (1995). *Centrally Commissioned Research Programme*. London: DH.

Department of Health (1995). *Centrally Commissioned Research Programme: Commissions in 1995*. London: DH.

Department of Health (1995). *Improving the Health of Mothers and Children: NHS Priorities for Research and Development*. London: DH.

Department of Health (1995). *Supporting Research and Development in the NHS: A Declaration of NHS Activity and Costs Associated with Research and Development, Initial Guidance*. London: DH.

HMSO (1994). *Supporting Research and Development in the NHS: The Report of a Task force led by Anthony Culyer*. London: HMSO.

Jones, R. (1993). 'Personal computer software for handling references from CD ROM and mainframe sources for scientific and medical reports'. *British Medical Journal*, Vol. 307, pp. 180–184.

Light, R.J., Pillemer, D.B. (1984). *Summing up: The Science of Reviewing Research*. Cambridge: M.A. Harvard University Press.

Locke, L.F., Spirduso, W.W., Silverman, S. (1993). *Proposals That Work: A Guide to Planning Dissertations and Grant Proposals*. London: Sage.

Lowe, H.J., Barnett, G.O. (1994). 'Understanding and using the Medical subject headings (MeSH) vocabulary to perform literature searches'. *Journal American Medical Association,* Vol. 271, No. 14, pp. 1103–1108.

Medical Research Council (1994). *Developing High Quality Proposals in Health Services Research.* London: MRC.

Medical Research Council (1995). *Research Developments Relevant to NHS Practice, Public Health and Health Departments Policy.* London: MRC.

Murphy, E., Spiegal, N., Kinmouth, A. (1992). 'Will you help with my research? Gaining access to primary health care settings and subjects'. *British Journal of General Practice,* Vol. 42, pp. 162–165.

Oxman, A., Sackett, D.L., Guyatt, G.H. (1993). 'Users' guides to the medical literature, How to get started'. *Journal American Medical Association,* Vol. 270, No. 17, pp. 2093–2095.

Pollit, C., Harrison, S., Hunter, D., Marnoch, G. (1990). 'No hiding place: On the discomforts of researching the contemporary policy process'. *Journal of Social Policy,* Vol. 19, No. 2, pp. 169–90.

Social Research Association (1994). *The SRA Guide to Good Practice for Commissioning Social Research.* Social Research Association, 116 Turney Road, London, SE21 7JJ.

Wisely, J., Haines, A. (1995). 'Commissioning a national programme of research and development on the interface between primary and secondary care'. *British Medical Journal,* Vol. 311, pp. 1080–1082.

Other

Altman, D.G. (1991). *Practical Statistics for Medical Research.* London: Chapman and Hall.

Berk, R.A., Rossi, P.H. (1990). *Thinking About Programme Evaluation.* London: Sage.

Department of Health (1991). *The Patients Charter, HPC1.* London: HMSO.

Department of Health (1992). *The Health of the Nation: A Strategy for Health in England, CM1986.* London: HMSO.

Department of Health (1993). *The Named Nurse, Midwife and Health Visitor.* London: DH.

Department of Health (1993). *Changing Childbirth, Part 1: Report of the Expert Maternity Group.* London: HMSO.

Department of Health (1994). *Standing Group on Health Technology: 1994 Report.* London: DH.

Department of Health (1995). *Report of the NHS Health Technology Assessment Programme.* London: DH.

Donabedian, A. (1980). *Explorations in Quality Assessment and Monitoring, Vol 1, The Definition Of Quality and Approaches to its Assessment.* Ann Arbor, Mich. Health Administration Press.

Fink, A. (1995). *The Survey Kit.* London: Sage.

Garcia, J. (1995). 'Continuity of care in context, What matters to women?'. In: Page, L. (Ed). *Effective Group Practice in Midwifery: Working With Women.* Oxford: Blackwell.

Goldberg, D. (1992). *The General Health Questionnaire.* NFER-NELSON.

Grady, K., Wallston, B.S. (1988). *Research in Health Care Settings.* London: Sage.

Hammersley, M., Atkinson, P. (1995). *Ethnography, Principles in Practice.* London: Routledge.

Herman, J.L. (1988). *Program Evaluation Kit.* London: Sage.

House of Commons (1992). *The Health Committee Second Report: Maternity Services, Vol 1.* (Chairman N. Winterton). London: HMSO.

House of Lords (1988). *Priorities in Medical Research, Select Committee on Science and Technology Session 1987–1988, Third Report, HL Paper 54.* London: HMSO.

Hunter, D. (1994). 'The aftermath of the NHS reforms'. In: Popay, J., Williams, G. (Eds). *Researching the People's Health.* London: Routledge.

Macfarlane, A., Mugford, M., Johnson, A., Garcia, J. (1995). *Counting the Changes in Childbirth: Trends and Gaps in National Statistics.* Oxford: National Perinatal Epidemiology Unit.

Murphy Black, T. (1992). 'Systems of midwifery care in use in Scotland'. *Midwifery,* Vol. 8, pp. 113–124.

Oakley, A. (1992). *Social Support and Motherhood.* Oxford: Basil Blackwell.

Ontario College of Midwives (1995). *Midwifery in Ontario.* Ontario: Ontario College of Midwives.

Roberts, H. (1990). *Women's Health Counts.* London: Routledge.

Roberts, H. (1992). *Women's Health Matters.* London: Routledge.

St. Leger, A.S., Schieden, H., Walsworth-Bell, J.P. (1992). *Evaluating Health Services Effectiveness.* Milton Keynes: Open University Press.

World Health Organization (1994). *Mother and Baby Package: Implementing Safe Motherhood in Countries.* Geneva: WHO.

Wraight, A., Ball, J., Seccombe, I., Stock, J. (1993). *Mapping Team Midwifery, A Report to the Department of Health, IMS Report series 242.* Sussex: Institute Manpower Studies.

Appendix

Database name	Description	Availability	Access
Cumulative Index to Nursing and Allied Health Literature (CINAHL)	American, nursing and paramedical	Online + CD ROM	Library
Biosis previews	Life sciences	CD ROM	Library
Medline	US National Library of Medicine Database + International Nursing Index + Dental Index	CD ROM + Online	Library
The Cochrane Library	Systematic reviews of randomized controlled trials of care in pregnancy and birth	Disc/ CD ROM	BMJ Publishing BMA House Tavistock Square London WC1H 9JR 0171 383 6185
BIDS Bath information and data service for Higher Education	Covers Science Citation index, Social Science Citation index, Arts and Humanities Index and Scientific and Technical Proceedings, Embase	Online subscription service	Library BIDS 01225 826074 Internet address http://www.bids.ac.uk
Sociofile	Sociological abstracts & social planning and policy development abstracts	CD ROM	Library
Psychlit	Psychological abstracts	CD ROM	Library
Embase	Biomedical science, health policy, abstracts	Online	Library
DHSS Data	Nursing Research abstracts Health and Social Services abstracts	Online	
Healthplan	Planning, administration, finance, management, manpower and insurance	CD ROM + Online	
HELMIS Health Management Information Service	Library database	CD ROM/ online	Nuffield Institute for Health Information Resource Centre (IRC)

Database of Social Research Methodology	Key references in social science methodology	CD ROM	Sage Publications Ltd 6 Bonhill Street London EC2A 4PU 0171 383 6185
RCN – Nurse ROM	RCN library journal database Journal titles from 1985	CD ROM	RCN library

NB: For suppliers of online databases ask librarian.

Table 1: Electronic databases and on-line searching

Name	Coverage	Access
Index Medicus	Mainly medical	
Index of Nursing Research	1968–1994 Research in progress and 'grey literature'	Superseded by DHSS - DATA
International Nursing Index (INI)	American, nursing, midwifery and health visiting	
Sociological Abstracts		
Psychological Abstracts		
DH Nursing Research Abstracts		
Applied Social Sciences Indexes and Abstracts	Sociology, psychology, health	
Health Service Abstracts		
Quality Assurance Abstracts		
Social Service Abstracts		
Nursing Citation Index		
Social Science Citation Index		
Current Contents: Clinical Practice		
Current Contents: Social and Behavioural Sciences		
Current literature on health services		DH
Midwifery Index		RCM Library

Table 2: Indexing, abstracting journals, current awareness bulletins

Name	Coverage	Address	Access
Changing Childbirth Team database of research in progress and practice initiatives	Database of ongoing NHS pilot projects and other research in the area	Changing Childbirth Team Health Care and Public Health Directorate NHS Executive Anglia and Oxford 6–12 Capital Drive Linford Wood Milton Keynes MK14 6QP 01908 844400	
Centre for Evidence Based Medicine	Systematic reviews & database of RCT's	Centre for Evidence Based Medicine Nuffield Department of Clinical Medicine Level 5 John Radcliffe Hospital Headington, Oxford OX3 9DU 01865 221321	http:// cebm.jr2. ox.ac.uk/
MIRIAD	Register of ongoing research in midwifery	MIRIAD Dept. Midwifery Studies University of Leeds 24 Hyde Terrace Leeds LS2 9LN 0113 2336872 [fax]	Published
National Research Register	Ongoing & planned research supported by NHS R & D and centrally commissioned programme	National Research Register Co-ordination Unit Vega Group Plc 2 Falcon Way Shire Park Welwyn Garden City Herts AL7 1TW 01707 391999	Access via Regional R & D Director Anne Dunlop NHS HQ Dept of Health Quarry House Quarry Hill Leeds LS2 7UE 0113 2546164
NHS Centre for Reviews & Dissemination	Systematic reviews + databases 1. Abstracts of reviews 2. NHS Economic evaluations 3. Full text reviews commissioned by CRD	University of York Heslington York YO1 5DD 01904 433634	Online CD ROM http://www. york.ac.uk/ inst/crd/ welcome.htm

MIDIRS, Midwifery Digest	Abstracts and critiqued research + original articles & database 480 journals covered	MIDIRS 9 Elmdale Road Clifton Bristol BS8 1SL 0800 581009	Published http://www. gn.apc.org/ midirs/services. htm
The UK Cochrane Centre	Systematic reviews of RCT's of health care. Co-ordinates international Cochrane collaboration	NHS R&D Programme Summertown Pavilion Middle Way Oxford OX2 7LG 01865 516300	Database published electronically http://hiru. mcmaster.ca/ cochrane/ default.htm
RCM Changing Childbirth Special Interest Group	Regular meetings	Ann Horne RCM English Board Office, 18th Floor Royal Exchange House Boar Lane Leeds LS1 5NY	

Table 3: Databases and networks of research in progress

Name	Coverage	Address
Midwifery home page	Gateway to international resources	http://medweb.bham.ac.uk/nursing/midwife/
HIRU quicklist Health Information Research Unit (USA) Evaluates health care information	Preventive care guidelines Guide to clinical preventive services Computers in patient education Clinical informatics Clinical practice guidelines	http://hiru.mcmaster.ca/fast.htm
SCHARR Sheffield Centre for Health and Health Related Research	Hypertext links to many other health related sites and produces guides to evidence based health care.	http://www.shef.ac.uk/uni/academic/R-Z/scharr/
NIH Consensus programme Information Service National Library Medicine Technology Assessment (US)	Consensus statements on medical technology assessment	http://text.nlm.nih.gov
Health Resources on the Web	Good starting site	http://www.ha.org.hk/qmh/qmrlist.html
US Library of Congress WWW home page		http://lcweb.loc.gov/homepage/lchp.html
Department of Health Home Page	Policy updates, press releases, R & D initiatives	http://www.open.gov.uk/doh/dhhome.htm
BMJ	Contents pages, abstracts and some articles	http://www.bmj.com/bmj/
Yahoo	Search engine com/health	http://www.yahoo.
WHO		http://www.who.ch
GP – UK home page	Good start site with many connections to other medical sites	http://www.ncl.ac.uk/~nphcare/GPUK/gpukhome.html
Bandolier – Evidence based medicine	Monthly journal Oxford Anglia NHS region	http://www.jr2.ox.ac.uk:80/bandolier/
South & West Region Health Care Libraries	NHSE S & W, R & D library Good start site	http://www.soton.ac.uk/~swhelu/
Midwifery Today online birth centre	Midwifery, pregnancy, breastfeeding. On line links worldwide, E-mail network	http://acnm.org/

Table 4: Internet resources

Name	Coverage	Address
Evidence-based health	Application of critical appraisal to problems in healthcare. List for teachers and professionals, to stimulate discussion and announce events	evidence-based-health on Mailbase
Health-econeval	Facilitates discussion on economic evaluation of health care, regular newsletter	health-econ-eval on Mailbase
Lis-medical	Intended for librarians but useful for research on effective healthcare	lis-medical on Mailbase
Public-health	Discussion forum and information resource for those working in epidemiology and public health	public-health on Mailbase

Table 5: Discussion lists

Index

The Index incorporates Authors (both personal and corporate), Titles (*in italics*) and Subject terms. If you want to look up general information on any topic, choose the page numbers indicated alongside the main entries. For more detailed information, choose the page numbers indicated alongside any appropriate sub–headings. Where several page numbers are listed, those **in bold type** represent a section of the book devoted to that topic. Cross–references can be used to guide you around the structure of the book and find topics of related interest.